Pregnancy and Birth in Russia

This book provides a theoretically and empirically grounded examination of the struggle for maternity care in contemporary Russia, framed by changes to the healthcare system and the roles of its participants after socialism. The chapters consider multiple perspectives and interactions between women and professionals and the structural and institutional pressures they face when striving for better conditions and treatment. Russian maternity care is characterized by the vivid mix of legacy of Soviet paternalism and medicalization, bureaucratic principles of state regulation (with high level of centralization and lack of professional autonomy) and global neoliberal tendencies. Maternity care professionals have to not only satisfy the growing needs and demands of women but also deal with increasing state regulative control, market demands and new professional standards of care. Navigating these multiple and various challenges, maternity providers have to perform in multiple roles to bridge the organizational gaps and inconsistencies. Thus, the field of struggle for good care becomes not only professional, but political one. Highlighting the opportunities and barriers for good care in the context of post-socialist Russia, this book will be of particular interest to medical anthropologists and sociologists as well as midwives and other health professionals.

Anna Temkina is Professor of Sociology, Chair in Public Health and Gender, and Co-Director of the Gender Studies Programme at the European University at Saint-Petersburg, Russia.

Anastasia Novkunskaya is a sociologist and an associate professor on qualitative health research at the Institute for Interdisciplinary Health Research at the European University at Saint-Petersburg, Russia.

Daria Litvina is a sociologist and research fellow at the Gender Studies Program and Institute for Interdisciplinary Health Research at European University at Saint-Petersburg, Russia.

Social Science Perspectives on Childbirth and Reproduction

Series editor: Robbie Davis-Floyd
Rice University, Houston, Texas

This series focuses on issues relating to childbirth and reproduction from social science perspectives. It includes single-authored, co-authored, or edited books concerned both with people's reproductive experiences and with birth practitioners such as midwives (both professional and traditional), obstetricians, nurses, doulas, and others. It seeks to provide new viewpoints on functional and sustainable birth models and the challenges to their creation and maintenance, as well as on obstetric violence, disrespect, and abuse and their root causes. Single-case or comparative ethnographies on birth and other reproductive issues are featured, from high-tech conceptions to normal pregnancy and birth, including reproductive politics and human-rights issues in reproduction worldwide.

Birthing Techno-Sapiens
Human-Technology Co-Evolution and the Future of Reproduction
Edited by Robbie Davis-Floyd

Negotiated Breastfeeding
Holistic Postpartum Care and Embodied Parenting
Caroline Chautems

Birth as an American Rite of Passage
Third Edition
Robbie Davis-Floyd

Doulas in Italy
The Emergence of a New Care Profession
Pamela Pasian

Pregnancy and Birth in Russia
The Struggle for "Good Care"
Anna Temkina, Anastasia Novkunskaya, and Daria Litvina

For more information about this series, please visit: www.routledge.com/Social-Science-Perspectives-on-Childbirth-and-Reproduction/book-series/SSPCR

Pregnancy and Birth in Russia

The Struggle for "Good Care"

Anna Temkina, Anastasia Novkunskaya, and Daria Litvina

Routledge
Taylor & Francis Group
LONDON AND NEW YORK

First published 2023
by Routledge
4 Park Square, Milton Park, Abingdon, Oxon OX14 4RN

and by Routledge
605 Third Avenue, New York, NY 10158

Routledge is an imprint of the Taylor & Francis Group, an informa business

British Library Cataloguing-in-Publication Data
A catalogue record for this book is available from the British Library

ISBN: 978-0-367-68895-0 (hbk)
ISBN: 978-0-367-68900-1 (pbk)
ISBN: 978-1-003-13953-9 (ebk)

DOI: 10.4324/9781003139539

Typeset in Sabon
by Apex CoVantage, LLC

Contents

Foreword

What constitutes "good" maternity care in Russia? This is one of the primary questions asked and answered in this outstanding book. We in the West know little about Russian maternity care, yet we should, as in its mirror we can see ourselves and our own technocratic birthways reflected and refracted, just as we can see the influence of the international movement for the humanization of birth – which, as Temkina, Novkunskaya and Litvina show, is slowly making inroads into Russian maternity care – in part due to international influences, in part to increased practitioner attention to the scientific evidence supporting humanistic childbirth and in part to childbearers' increasing demands for humanized care.

While these authors acknowledge that the massive overuse of technomedical interventions that characterizes birth in Russia also characterizes birth in most other countries, they also demonstrate that Russian birthways carry their own unique set of twist and turns, beginning with the move from Soviet to post-Soviet maternity care and continuing on to the neoliberal marketing and consumerization of pregnancy and birth in Russia. It is impossible to understand the current obstetric management of Russian birth without first understanding what preceded it in the Soviet period, during which birth was treated in an industrialized, conveyor-belt style undergirded by patriarchy, paternalism, total State control and a de-humanized treatment style specific to Russia called *khamstvo*. This term indexes rudeness, verbal and sometimes physical abuse of women during labor and birth, and women as helpless and passive recipients of this rudely doled out treatment; it conveys a general ethos of "women-unfriendly" maternity services. As these authors explain in detail, during the Soviet, *khamstvo* era of Russian childbirth, childbearing women had absolutely no choice regarding where, how and with whom they would give birth, nor in how they would be treated. This maternity care management, now called "the System" by both patients and practitioners, was considered both normal and normative in practitioner's and childbearers' minds. And the System is equated with the State – the national government of Russia, from Putin on down.

Today, childbirth and maternity care in Russia are changing, moving from the older Soviet model of *khamstvo* to a post-Soviet model characterized by the tensions among neoliberal market reforms, the still-rigid control of Russian State bureaucracies, and the new consumerist style. Obstetricians and other maternity care practitioners find themselves trapped "between the rock and the anvil" – as the Russian saying goes – the "rock" being the State (a.k.a. "the System") and the "anvil" being women's new consumer orientations toward achieving "good care." As efforts at humanization have crept in, providers have found themselves obliged to be polite and to smile – behaviors that had previously been very far outside of their patient treatment repertoire. Some enjoy and appreciate this more humanistic approach, while others sometimes long to go back to "the way it was," when practitioners had total control over perinatal care and childbearing women had none.

As I see it, this book addresses three primary struggles: (1) the perceptions, opinions and experiences of Russian maternity care providers – most especially obstetricians – as they struggle to provide "good care" as they understand it; (2) those of the childbearers who struggle to achieve good care as they perceive it; and (3) the experiences of the authors as ethnographers, who had to struggle to be accepted by the staff of the primary hospital in which they conducted most of the extensive ethnographic research on which this book is based. I will address each of these struggles in turn.

The Struggles of Obstetricians and Other Maternity Care Providers

The status of obstetricians in Russia is quite different from that in other countries, in that Russian obstetricians have little to no autonomy, as they are subjected to the rules and regulations laid down by the State/the System, by the institutions in which they work and by different departments within those institutions. Thus, their "birthscape"[1] is fraught with contradictions, as these regulations and rules often conflict with and/or contradict each other, leaving obstetricians, midwives, nurses – and hospital administrators – to try to figure out which rules to follow and when and to negotiate the best ways to provide good care that will not subject them or their hospitals to State sanctions. Add to this a lack of necessary resources and sufficient staff and the "burden" of having to try to satisfy patients' newly consumeristic demands, and the (predictable) result is practitioners who are overstressed, overworked and overburdened – a perfect recipe for their not-infrequent regressions to *khamstvo*-style care – in which they can perpetrate their frustrations onto vulnerable birthing bodies.

The Struggles of Childbearing Women for "Good" Care

Having heard multiple horror stories from their mothers and grandmothers about Soviet-style care, and empowered by the relatively recent turn toward regarding health and maternity care as commodities that can be bought and paid for (within a System in which all care is free – unless women want options), today's young and affluent Russian women often struggle to find paid private services that allow them to choose both their hospital and their birth practitioners – specifically their obstetrician and midwife. Such women want the continuity of care and the physical and emotional comfort such private, for-pay services promise to provide, and often do. Yet, unlike many childbearers living in high resource countries who create elaborate birth plans spelling out their expectations and desires, these affluent Russian women see their agency and control in choosing their practitioners and place of birth, after which they are happy to give up agency and control to those practitioners during labor and birth, firmly believing that "the doctor knows best." For Russian maternity care, and Russian society in general, are based not so much on patriarchy as on *paternalism* – in which childbearers expect the paternalistic State, maternity care facilities as State institutions, and obstetricians as State representatives to have the authority to manage the perinatal process in multiple ways.

Those childbearers – the majority – who cannot afford to pay for more personalized, humanistic care adopt strategies of navigation and negotiation, using their social networks to find doctors willing to establish some sort of personal relationship with them – often only to find that a birth that was proceeding well is "ruined" when the shift changes and *khamstvo*-style practitioners take over. Thus, there are websites filled with Soviet-style "horror stories" of contemporary births, and many women file formal complaints with government agencies, which hospital administrators then have to deal with, as they are required by law to do. This adds to their already huge volume of paperwork and generates anger against those "spoiled" and "selfish" women who complain about practitioners, who in their minds were doing their best to provide "good care."

The Struggles of "Sociologists in White"

In the large tertiary care center in which the authors conducted most of the long-term ethnographic research on which this book is based, which they simply call "the Hospital," they found themselves constantly struggling to explain and to justify their presence to each department and to each practitioner with whom they interacted. "Who are you, and what are you doing here?" were constant refrains. Eventually, to better fit in, they began to wear white coats, which made them look and feel to hospital personnel like "one of us" instead of "the Others" – a process that ultimately resulted in them being called "*our* sociologists" as staff members began to take pride in the work of these "sociologists in white." It seems to me that their interviewing process was to some extent therapeutic for those interviewed – those staff members had never before been *listened to* with such interest, intensity and appreciation. To establish trust, the authors conducted these interviews before they began observing practitioners' work. They also established trust by presenting some of their early research results at a conference for staff that was held by the hospital, at which their presentation was well-received – illustrating the importance of reciprocity in ethnography.

In addition to its comprehensive overview of Russian maternity care and the rapid changes it is undergoing, this unique book provides a comprehensive understanding of what social scientists can accomplish – and how they can accomplish it – when they work in a biomedical field site. Its authors illustrate the horizons of *the ethnographic possible*, which include the importance of gaining trust, the need to have patience for the process and the intricacies of navigating a bureaucracy so complex that I am amazed that they could make such comprehensible sense out of the often seemingly senseless practices and procedures that were daily performed. At first out of place in that huge Hospital, these authors found ways to create space and place for themselves within its walls. Thus, this book, in addition to informing its readers about the ever-changing state of Russian maternity care, also teaches us much about ethnography – what it is and how to do it within a generally closed biomedical facility that rarely takes kindly to "outsiders."

In sum, as this book shows, Russia is a country in transition from socialism to certain, limited forms of capitalism, and from Soviet-style maternity care to more humanized approaches. Certainly, with this book and with, over time, their multiple presentations of the results of their research to hospital staff, these "sociologists in white" have made major contributions toward that highly worthwhile end – showing that social scientists have much to offer biomedical practitioners, and vice versa. As these authors explain, "The field changed us, and we changed the field." It is my hope that this book will find a large readership and that at least some of those readers will also engage in the process of creating change "from within."

Robbie Davis-Floyd
Author of *Birth as an American Rite of Passage*
(1992, 2003, 2022)
Austin, Texas
October 2021

Acknowledgments

This book could not have been completed without invaluable help by Robbie Davis-Floyd, who not only endorsed our book proposal and carefully reviewed all the chapters of the manuscript but inspired for some analytical conclusions and provoked our sociological imagination.

We would like to acknowledge the financial assistance of our study, provided by the Russian Science Foundation (Project No. 19-78-10128) and the Professorship on gender and health, hosted at the European University at Saint-Petersburg. We could not have collected all the data and conduct institutional ethnography of the Hospital without this valuable maintenance. In particular we are deeply grateful to Ekaterina Borozdina, the head of the project "*Patient centered care in Russian healthcare: organizational challenges and professionals' opportunities*," who supported our fieldwork and commented on the drafts of our chapters, giving insightful feedback, which moved us forward.

We also thank our (unknown) reviewers of our book proposal, who gave us chance to proceed with the idea of the manuscript. There have been many other colleagues, who created a favorable environment for our study, endlessly discussing chapters' drafts, giving feedback on the papers, presented at the conferences and working seminars. Among them we are particularly grateful to Michele Rivkin-Fish and Julia Lerner for their careful reading and strict but fair criticism of our first thoughts about different emotional styles in Russian maternity care; to Anna Ozhiganova, who kindly agreed to review our chapter on professional agency; to Alena Ledeneva and Petra Matijevic, from the "Global Informality Project" for their comments on Russian practice of *khamstvo*.

We have had the great opportunity to work together with Elena Zdravomyslova, Elena Bogdanova, Alia Nizamova, Anastasia Ugarova, Maria Pirogovskaya, Anna Klepikova, Anna Altukhova, and Olga Tkach at the Program of "Gender Studies" and Program of "Social Studies of Health and Medicine" at the European University at Saint-Petersburg (EUSP). Multiple discussions and events with them have considerably shaped the direction of our study, sharpened our methodological reflection and navigated us both empirically and analytically. We also would like to express our thanks to other colleagues from EUSP and Saint-Petersburg Association of Sociologists (SPAS) for organizing fruitful discussions and their valuable comments on some parts of the book, critique and ideas on improvement. We thank all the interviewers and transcribers, who participated in the projects and helped us to collect and handle the data.

We would like to acknowledge invaluable contribution to our study by midwives and nurses from Russian Association of Medical Nurses (RAMS), especially Julia Agapova and Viktoria Kuznetsova, who have become more than our interlocutors and colleagues, as they inspired us to discover professional agency in Russian maternity care.

We feel a sense of profound gratitude to all our interlocutors, who agreed to participate in the study in different maternity hospitals and other facilities in different cities in Russia: childbearing women and their partners, obstetricians and other physicians, midwives, nurses, psychologists, other professionals, administrators and organizers of public health and maternity care. Although we still cannot mention the name of the Hospital, we are deeply grateful to the Hospital's Administration for their interest in sociology, trust to researchers and the very possibility to conduct the research. We also thank all the physicians, nurses, midwives, technical workers and patients of the Hospital for letting us dive into the network of their communication and learn so much about the complicated world of maternity care.

Note

1 As far as I know, "birthscape" is a term that was coined by one of my interns, Julie Post. I thank her for allowing me to use it in my work.

Chapter 1

Introducing the struggle for "good care" in Russian maternity care

Transformations in maternity care have been under scrutiny in the social sciences worldwide. The aim of this book is to enrich this knowledge with evidence from the post-Soviet context, which not only is subject to global tendencies, but also has some unique traits that call for special attention. This book will explain how and why things are different (or similar) in Russian maternity care compared to Western countries, in order to provide new perspectives on understanding maternity care globally. We focus on maternity hospitals – the only legal sites for maternity care provision in Russia.

In this book, we address global feminist debates regarding childbirth experiences, women's empowerment (Crossley, 2007; Sandall et al., 2009; Witz, 2013; Malacrida & Boulton, 2014; Rothman, 2014; Feeley & Thomson, 2016), ethics of care (Mol, 2008, 2002; Brodwin, 2013), and the effects of health and maternity care reforms triggered by neoliberalism and consumerism in relation to healthcare institutions' design and alterations (Dent, 2006; Clarke et al., 2006, 2007; Berry, 2010; Timmermans & Oh, 2010; Numerato et al., 2012; Fotaki, 2014; Bell & Green, 2016; Mercille, 2018). We also introduce our research on the struggle for "good care" in Russian maternity care as a contribution to the discussions on patient-centered (or women-centered) care (Rivkin-Fish, 2005; Ozhiganova, 2009; Borozdina, 2016; Borozdina & Novkunskaya, 2019; Temkina, 2019; Temkina & Rivkin-Fish, 2020; Litvina et al., 2020) and on political-economic transformations after socialism, which we develop by applying a neo-institutional analytical framework to the analysis of healthcare institutions and their changes (Lawrence et al., 2009; Muzio et al., 2013; Cloutier et al., 2015; Thornton et al., 2015; Zilber, 2016). This is especially important as we still lack relevant comprehensive knowledge about recent transformations in childbirth in this context, especially those taking place in Russian maternity hospitals (with the exception of overall research conducted by Rivkin-Fish (2005) from the 1990s to the 2000s).

Many social scientists critique the growth of managerialism and marketization in healthcare, as they challenge both patients' rights and agency and practitioners' professional autonomy. In Russia, these processes are shaped

DOI: 10.4324/9781003139539-1

in a particular way, in which the notion of "good care" is not a constant issue, but rather a perpetual, mostly invisible, negotiation between various actors, including women, their families, physicians, midwives, nurses, hospital administrators and State officials, all of whom have different spheres of interest and agendas (financial, professional, political), and strive toward different practices of medicalized care. The interactions among social actors with differing ideologies and ideals of "good care" comprise the main focus of this book, in which we nuance the relationships between childbearing women and maternity care providers. We explore their interactions as framed both by practices that stem from the Soviet era and by the changes made in recent decades.

In spite of humanizing changes, childbearing women in Russia, as elsewhere, cannot count on having unconditional access to women-centered care, nor can maternity care practitioners (who would like to provide such care) gain the necessary institutional support to provide it. We seek herein to get at why women-centered care is still problematic in post-Soviet Russia in spite of numerous reforms implemented to improve maternity care, starting in the 1990s and reinforced from 2000 to the present.

Beginning with Jordan (1978), multiple studies of childbirth have been conducted in numerous social and cultural contexts. As feminist critics argue, the conditions of childbirth in different contexts depend on cultural attitudes toward birth, the structures of maternity care, the interplay of different attendants and providers and also on women's agency and their empowerment (or lack thereof) (Benoit et al., 2005; Sandall et al., 2009). All these preconditions are quite specific in the post-Soviet context, especially in terms of the particularities of gender relations, healthcare institutions and reforms, the socio-structural positions of childbearing women, practitioners' positions in the maternity care system and how new reforms are changing these positions.

Problematic issues in Russian maternity care

We address problematic issues in Russian maternity care via four major topics: (1) patriarchy and paternalism in Russian maternity care; (2) the hybridization of post-Soviet health and maternity care via marketization and neoliberal reforms; (3) women positioning and women-centered care in post-Soviet Russia; and (4) the effects of reforms and the Soviet legacy on practitioners' routines.

Patriarchy and paternalism in Russian maternity care

First, we note that a patriarchal gender system is one of the key structural preconditions organizing global maternity care. The gendered dimensions of social control and power in the male-dominated field of obstetrics have long been subjects of feminist criticism and reassessments of reproductive health (Davis-Floyd, 2001, 2003; Witz, 2013). The gendered system of predominantly male doctors and female midwives and nurses that often characterized Western obstetrics until the 1970s was different in Russia, as the majority of obstetricians there (and of physicians in general) are women (Schecter, 2000; Riska, 2001). Hence, lack of "good care" cannot be explained by patriarchy only. In this book, we problematize the basic assumptions of previous feminist studies on women-centered care as struggling with patriarchy. The mostly female physicians in Russia try to maintain their medicalized power and authoritative positions in the context of ongoing healthcare reforms (Temkina, 2019). Citizens' rights of women in feminized maternity care rarely become an issue of public debate and the feminist agenda in Russia. Yet although patriarchy does not dominate the Russian maternity care system, it *is* dominated by paternalism – a system positing that those in authority "know best" and that may be outwardly benevolent, but often in a condescending or controlling way. The primary struggles that we address herein lie in the articulations and clashes between the government-controlled paternalistic system and the personal strivings of both practitioners and women toward "good maternity care."

The hybridization of the post-Soviet health and maternity care system: marketization and neoliberal reforms

Second, we address the particular post-Soviet institutionalized practices of healthcare characterized simultaneously by overmedicalization of childbirth (as elsewhere around the world, childbearing women are mostly treated as patients, not active agents in biomedical hospitals); paternalistic State dominance in the field of maternity care; the ongoing transformations of key social institutions; and the developing consumer markets. The shift from the socialist *Semashko* healthcare system (which we will describe further later on) to a neoliberal system facilitated both managerial overregulation in terms of increasing State control and new market demands affecting the standards of care. We conceptualize the post-Soviet systems of healthcare and maternity care as *hybrids* of the legacy of Soviet bureaucratic paternalism and new neoliberal reforms, which enhance managerialism and marketization in medical settings. Thus, the defining peculiarity of the Russian case is the extremely strong role of the State in institutionalizing certain practices of childbirth, as multiple State bodies limit health providers' autonomy, subordinate medical professionals to bureaucratic needs and prioritize statistical and economic indicators of their work. This centralized, top-down organization of ruling relations restricts the possibilities for women-centered care as it puts the State's interests in the center.

The design, arrangement and provision of maternity care in Russia are shaped by three key features: (1) its continuance of certain Soviet principles;

(2) its perpetual and inconsistent neoliberal transformations over recent decades; and (3) as a result, its institutional inconsistencies. Different organizational logics have led to unintentional consequences: multiple gaps, discontinuities and uncertainties in maternity care; the vulnerability of women as dependent on maternity care providers; and the vulnerability of the latter as dependent on both patients (for their income) and healthcare managers. Such preconditions shape the positions of childbearing women and practitioners, who want to receive and provide "good care," but must negotiate and struggle to achieve it.

Women-centered care in post-Soviet Russia

Third, feminist researchers for decades have argued that childbearing women want to participate in decision-making; they want to have better conditions and a less medicalized approach to childbirth (Lazarus, 1994) with strong focus on their needs. Women-centered care is oriented on choice and on humanistic and holistic models of care (Davis-Floyd, 2001, 2003, 2018) that take into account both clinical and psychosocial aspects of the childbearing process, provide continuity of care and advocate a variety of approaches to (low-risk) pregnancies and births. Scholars argue that women struggle for recognition of their agency and have become more empowered in childbirth, which consequently in some places has become less medicalized and more egalitarian. Therefore, maternity care, by virtue of feminist and activist movements, has reached the avant-garde of healthcare transformations in some high-resource countries, such as New Zealand, the Netherlands, Norway, Denmark, Japan and a few others (see Davis-Floyd & Cheyney, 2019). Russia is clearly not one of these. In this book, we present the positions of women in the particular post-Soviet context, defined by vigilance toward feminism, limited opportunities for voicing one's positions, and consequent disengagement from activism.

Some women can benefit from neoliberal reforms in healthcare, but these reforms are criticized globally as exaggerating the positive effects on patients' choice, since the resources poured into enhanced choice for some women (white, middle-class) can also lead to the growth of inequality and decrease access to care for other women (Indigenous, of color, low resource) (Clarke et al., 2006; Dent, 2006; Clarke et al., 2007; Ward & England, 2007; Fotaki, 2006, 2014; Gabe et al., 2015).

In Russia, childbearing women had little or no choice in the late Soviet system of maternity care; they had to submit to the monitoring of their pregnancies and give birth in certain State medical institutions without any choice or alternative. The particular hospital was predetermined for every woman according to her place of residence. Maternity hospitals were closed organizations, similar to "total institutions," with no access for relatives, no possibilities to bring personal belongings (including underwear), shared delivery rooms for several women simultaneously giving birth, overcrowded postnatal wards, staff shortages and overburdened and rude personnel.

Maternity care in Russia is perpetually changing, and more demands for "good care" are emerging. When in 2006 childbearing women received the possibility to choose their maternity hospital, it was only a prepaid option. Since then, this choice has become covered by mandatory health insurance and is available to every pregnant woman. Now maternity hospitals have to compete for patients, improve conditions and offer better services. The possibilities provided by neoliberal tendencies have become a relief for post-Soviet women. Instead of being obedient patients with no choice, women have become assertive consumers. In other words, the changing political and economic contexts have created a new type of patient-consumer.

Childbearing women as patient-consumers spend a lot of time and effort in seeking to organize and negotiate "good care" during pregnancy and childbirth in medical settings, carefully making the "right choice" among available options. This consequently led to changes in their style of interactions with medical providers, who in turn became more polite and attentive. Such changes in the emotional aspects of care (Temkina et al., 2021) have of course been beneficial for women. However, their choices are still limited – there is no other legal option to give birth than in hospitals (which are mostly State-funded) with an obstetrician and an assistant midwife, as homebirth and independent midwifery practice are illegal in Russia. Thus, this shift does not necessarily empower women as social actors and does not challenge existing power relations, where still both (mostly female) obstetricians and childbearing women continue to be in hierarchical relations subordinated to paternalistic State regulation. Women can still find themselves vulnerable and helpless during delivery in Russian maternity hospitals.

The effects of hybridization of maternity care and market reforms on practitioners

Fourth, as feminist critics argue, women's and newborns' well-being depends on professionals' knowledge and vision of maternity care. Providers, in their turn, experience the effects of market reforms, which alter their practices and the organization of healthcare in a variety of ways (Sandall et al., 2009). Critics tend to say that under increasing managerialism and consumerism, the work of practitioners has become more standardized and less autonomous, and they have become more profit-oriented, and this, in turn, negatively affects the quality of care provided (Ibid.; Numerato et al., 2012; Bevort & Suddaby, 2015; Reay & Jones, 2016).

Healthcare providers' situation in Russia is different in this respect. In Soviet Russia, obstetricians and other physicians never had professional autonomy in the sense that "Western" physicians used to have at that time.

The State had a monopoly on healthcare provision, which was free, but undermined choice both for care receivers and providers. At that time, medical professions were socially "respectable," but the salaries of healthcare providers were equalized and low. Their social prestige was rooted not in professional autonomy, but in their position as State employees, which supplied them with exclusive rights to be the only gatekeepers to limited collective goods (healthcare services).

Currently, Russian obstetricians and other physicians are in an ambivalent position. On the one hand, with the emergence of private health and maternity care sector, they have received more possibilities for professional development. On the other hand, their autonomy is still limited by the State and also by market demands. Nowadays, hospitals from many sectors of healthcare (including maternity care) are expected to attract patients, who can now make their own choices. The market orientation of State-funded facilities combined with its rigid bureaucratic regulations has multidirectional consequences for physicians, especially in maternity care.

Healthcare practitioners feel themselves deprived of professional autonomy and former high status and perceive that as a threat to their professional identity. Physicians often express nostalgic feelings about the previous respect they received from obedient patients (e.g., childbearing women) who unconditionally followed their instructions. Providers nowadays have to satisfy growing patient requests and demands and provide good service, while dealing with new professional tasks and standards of care. Physicians face more demands for professional competencies and for the emotional labor – they have to be more effective, service-oriented, polite, and attentive to women's requirements – in both private and State-funded segments of healthcare. These are essential in maternity care. Obstetricians, neonatologists, nurses and midwives try to provide the best care they can, but their autonomy and possibilities are limited by numerous, often contradictory, bureaucratic and economic requirements imposed by different State-controlling bodies. As a result, maternity care providers have to continually renegotiate their professional roles under these multiple pressures.

An overview of the contents of this book

In subsequent chapters, we discuss both the theoretical and empirical results of our findings, which relate to healthcare reforms, the hybrid system of Russian maternity care, women's experiences and maternity care providers' perspectives. In Chapter 2, we describe our data (which is also presented in greater detail in the Appendices) and reflect on our peculiar scholars' position in the ethnographic field as an ongoing process of renegotiation among different actors. The primary site of our research is a highly technologically developed and well-equipped perinatal hospital in a large Russian city offering all kinds of perinatal care – from assisted reproductive technologies (ARTs) and obstetrics to delivery and infant surgery. This choice of empirical site gave us the possibility to investigate the whole complex of organizational interactions among patients, maternity care providers and hospital administration in different departments. In this chapter, we also take a reflexive look at ourselves as researchers in interactions with maternity care providers.

Chapter 3 of this book consists of analyses of the historical, ideological and structural conditions shaping the current system of maternity care in Russia, with particular attention to the hybridization of State paternalism and marketization and the consequent emergence of institutional uncertainties. Maternity care, as a system associated with demographic issues and pronatalist concerns, has become symbolically significant to the authorities, provoking additional efforts to redesign the provision, regulation and arrangement of maternity services. The recent transformations in Russian maternity care, which are still framed as a State priority in a top-down manner, represent a special case for investigation, owing to their scale, speed and volatility. We describe the path of the State reforms in 1990s–2010s and other societal processes that have shaped the transformation of post-Soviet maternity care during the last three decades: decentralization in the 1990s; demographic ideological concerns in the mid-2000s; and centralization, also from the mid-2000s. We analyze how these result in multiple contradictions. Different principles of regulation have been developed in the studied field, evoking practical discrepancies that will be addressed in this chapter. We will analyze the trajectory of childbearing women as demonstrating the discontinuity of maternity care and practical issues in maternity hospital as demonstrating contradictory ruling logics and inconsistency in organization of care. These issues comprise the context of our further discussion on childbearing women's (Chapter 4) and maternity care providers (Chapter 5) positions within the System of maternity care and their negotiations for "good care."

In Chapter 4, we summarize our empirical findings on women's agency, their demands and attitudes toward maternity care, and their discontents. We show that young Russian women have become more assertive in comparison to previous generations and claim their right to more consumer-oriented services. This shift proceeds under the influence of neoliberal ideology, which combines neo-traditionalist ideas about motherhood with consumer-oriented individualism. In seeking "good care," women want to avoid the Soviet-type emotional style of *khamstvo* (rudeness). They try to make the "right choice" of providers and to create trustful relationships with them in order to get more personalized care. However, hospital conditions and the behavior of maternity care practitioners are often far from meeting women's expectations. When women have unexpected clinical complications or do not receive the expected level of comfort or emotional support, they feel themselves suffering victims of "obstetric aggression." Such women often mistrust providers and suspect that they act against their interests, using unreasonable clinical practices, poor coordination during birth, ignorance and disregard. Women also pay attention to communication style, emotional support and comfort level. Inappropriate communication and emotional style often become bases for discontent and for the increasing number of complaints to different State bodies and online.

Chapter 5 addresses new and "old" actors in maternity care and their negotiations around "good care." The multifaceted notions of "good care" are formulated by the State-determined standards and requirements; new market and consumer demands; and new actors in the field of maternity care. The neoliberal policies create new spaces for some professional groups to offer their practices in maternity hospitals; these can be independent midwives, doulas and perinatal psychologists. Hospital practitioners have to fulfill different roles in order to meet new expectations and demands – acting as clinicians, service providers, State bureaucrats – and must apply various techniques to cope with the inconsistencies and challenges that they face in their daily professional routines. Maternity care providers cope with these challenges and conflicting requirements by applying systematic "manual management." In other words, providers constantly negotiate with each other to solve numerous routine and urgent problems when formal rules are unhelpful and contradictory. Meeting all the formal requirements and navigating patients through organizational routines under inconsistent rules leads to practitioners' overload with duties, responsibilities and patients' informal demands. In order to meet different patients' demands and prevent complaints, they have to apply notable amounts of emotional labor, which makes them feel like service workers rather than high-ranking professionals. We show that emotional styles are entangled with multiple modes of care and emphasize that these are now changing: the formerly taken-for-granted Soviet rudeness (*khamstvo*) and disregard in maternity care are challenged by new professional standards and consumers' demands for newly supportive care that include courtesy and smiles. As the result, the professional group of maternity care practitioners (first of all obstetricians), who are socially considered to be in a powerful position, find themselves under overall control and are indeed limited in their possibilities to provide "good care."

Finally, in Chapter 6, we analyze the civic struggle of professionals with the neoliberal and paternalistic tendencies that make professional issues become political ones (in ways similar to the feminist "personal as political" agenda). This chapter is devoted to the civic struggles of professionals with the neoliberal and paternalistic tendencies that make professional issues into political ones (in terms of the feministic understanding of "the personal as political"). We apply feminist and strategic action field approaches to analyze new initiatives in maternity care from NGOs, professional unions and the grassroot activities of hospital midwives and nurses. These actors are "challengers," who contribute to the improvement of maternity care and to the empowerment of both practitioners and patients. They initiate struggles for more professional autonomy and better care; the repertoire of their strategies includes semi-legal practices outside and inside maternity facilities; educational and lawmaking work in professional associations; public protest voicing; and the creation of an infrastructure that would close the gaps in the State's healthcare system. Nowadays *professional* issues in Russia are becoming fields of *political* actions, while the professionals empower themselves by challenging existing rules and the institutional order.

In our Conclusion (Chapter 7), we return to the questions we are answering throughout the book: What constitutes "good maternity care" in Russia in the 21st century? Why, after numerous reforms and improvements, does Russian maternity care continue to underserve the interests of its providers and receivers? How do actors in the field of maternity care struggle for "good care" in their routine interactions within maternity hospitals and beyond? And how does "political" correspond with "professional" in this field of struggle? We formulate the six main conclusions we have come to in our research on structural issues in maternity care, changes in the positions of its providers and recipients, System challengers, the particularities of ethnographic study in maternity care facilities and the feminist vision. As a result of our research, we come to the conclusion that "good care" in Russian maternity hospitals is not a project of "women's empowerment," but rather a complex of negotiations among different actors with limited opportunities. We argue that universal ("Western") trends in both gender relations and women-centered care as the basic assumptions of previous research appear to be more nuanced and more diverse globally when we take into account post-Soviet maternity care.

References

Bell, K., & Green, J. (2016). On the perils of invoking neoliberalism in public health critique. *Critical Public Health*, 26(3), 239–243.

Benoit, C., Wrede, S., Bourgaeult, I., Sandall, J., De Vries, R., & Teijlingen, E. R. (2005). Understanding the social organization of maternity care systems: Midwifery as a touchstone. *Sociology of Health and Illness*, 27(6), 722–737.

Berry, N. S. (2010). *Unsafe Motherhood: Mayan Maternal Mortality and Subjectivity in Post-War Guatemala* (Vol. 21). New York and Oxford: Berghahn Books.

Bevort, F., & Suddaby, R. (2015). Scripting professional identities: How individuals make sense of contradictory institutional logics. *Journal of Professions and Organization*, 3(1), 17–38.

Borozdina, E. (2016). Professional care in maternity hospitals, benefits and challenges. *Zhurnal Issledovanii Sotsialnoi Politiki [The Journal of Social Policy Studies]*, 14, 479–492 (In Russian).

Borozdina, E., & Novkunskaya, A. (2019). The patients' perspective on institutional logics in Russian maternity care. *Zhurnal Issledovanii Sotsialnoi Politiki [The Journal of Social Policy Studies]*, 17(3), 439–452.

Brodwin, P. (2013). *Everyday Ethics: Voices from the Front Line of Community Psychiatry*. Berkeley, Los Angeles, and London: University of California Press.

Clarke, J., Newman, J., Smith, N., Vidler, E., & Westmarland, L. (2007). *Creating Citizen-Consumers: Changing Publics and Changing Public Services*. London: Sage.

Clarke, J., Smith, N., & Vidler, E. (2006). The indeterminacy of choice: Political, policy and organizational implications. *Social Policy and Society*, 5(3), 327–336.

Cloutier, C., Denis, J. L., Langley, A., & Lamothe, L. (2015). Agency at the managerial interface: Public sector reform as institutional work. *Journal of Public Administration Research and Theory*, 26(2), 259–276.

Crossley, M. (2007). Childbirth, complications and the illusion of 'choice': A case study. *Feminism and Psychology*, 17(4), 543–563.

Davis-Floyd, R. E. (2001). The technocratic, humanistic, and holistic paradigms of childbirth. *International Journal of Gynecology & Obstetrics*, 75(S5).

Davis-Floyd, R. E. (2003). *Birth as American Rite of Passage* (2nd ed.). Berkeley: University of California Press.

Davis-Floyd, R. E. (2018). Open and closed knowledge systems, the 4 stages of cognition, and the cultural management of birth. *Frontiers in Sociology*, 3, 23. https://doi.org/10.3389/fsoc2018.2018.0023.

Davis-Floyd, R. E., & Cheyney, M. (2019). *Birth in Eight Cultures*. Long Grove, IL: Waveland Press.

Dent, M. (2006). Patient choice and medicine in healthcare. *Public Management Review*, 8(3), 449–462.

Feeley, C., & Thomson, G. (2016). Tensions and conflicts in 'choice': Womens' experiences of freebirthing in the UK. *Midwifery*, 41, 16–21.

Fotaki, M. (2006). Users' perceptions of healthcare reforms: Quality of care and patient rights in four regions in the Russian Federation. *Social Science & Medicine*, 63, 1637–1647.

Fotaki, M. (2014). Can consumer choice replace trust in the National Health Service in England? Towards developing an affective psychosocial conception of trust in healthcare. *Sociology of Health & Illness*, 36(8), 1276–1294.

Gabe, J., Harley, K., & Calnan, M. (2015). Healthcare choice: Discourses, perceptions, experiences and practices. *Current Sociology*, 63(5), 623–635.

Jordan, B. (1978). *Birth in Four Cultures: A Crosscultural Investigation of Childbirth in Yucatan, Holland, Sweden, and the United States*. Montreal and St. Albans: Eden Press.

Lawrence, T. B., Suddaby, R., & Leca, B. (2009). *Institutional Work: Actors and Agency in Institutional Studies of Organizations*. Cambridge: Cambridge University Press.

Lazarus, E. (1994). What do women want?: Issues of choice, control, and class in pregnancy and childbirth. *Medical Anthropology Quarterly*, 8(1), 25–46.

Litvina, D., Novkunskaya, A., & Temkina, A. (2020). Multiple vulnerabilities in medical settings: Invisible suffering of doctors. *Societies*, 10(1), 5.

Malacrida, C., & Boulton, T. (2014). The best laid plans? Women's choices, expectations and experiences in childbirth. *Health*, 18(1), 41–59.

Mercille, J. (2018). Neoliberalism and healthcare: The case of the Irish nursing home sector. *Critical Public Health*, 28(5), 546–559.

Mol, A. (2002). *The Body Multiple: Ontology in Medical Practice*. Durham, NC: Duke University Press.

Mol, A. (2008). *The Logic of Care: Health and the Problem of Patient Choice*. Abingdon, Oxon: Routledge.

Muzio, D., Brock, D. M., & Suddaby, R. (2013). Professions and institutional change: Towards an institutionalist sociology of the professions. *Journal of Management Studies*, 50(5), 699–721.

Numerato, D., Salvatore, D., & Fattore, G. (2012). The impact of management on medical professionalism: A review. *Sociology of Health & Illness*, 34(4), 626–644.

Ozhiganova, A. (2009). Sovremennye perinatal'nye kul'tury: tradicionnaja i al'ternativnaja modeli [Modern perinatal cultures: Traditional and alternative models]. In *Polevye materialy Instituta jetnologii i antropologii RAN, 2006 [Field Materials of the Institute of Ethnology and Anthropology RAS, 2006]* (pp. 63–82). Moscow: IEA RAS (In Russian).

Reay, T., & Jones, C. (2016). Qualitatively capturing institutional logics. *Strategic Organization*, 14(4), 441–454.

Riska, E. (2001). *Medical Careers and Feminist Agendas: American, Scandinavian and Russian Women Physicians*. New York: Aldine de Gruyter,

Rivkin-Fish, M. (2005). *Women's Health in Post-Soviet Russia: The Politics of Intervention*. Bloomington: Indiana University Press.

Rothman, B. (2014). Pregnancy, birth and risk: An introduction. *Health, Risk & Society*, 16(1), 1–6.

Sandall, J., Benoit, C., Wrede, S., Murray, S. F., van Teijlingen, E. R., & Westfall, R. (2009). Social service professional or market expert? *Current Sociology*, 57(4), 529–553.

Schecter, K. (2000). The politics of healthcare in Russia: The feminization of medicine and other obstacles to professionalism. In M. G. Field & J. L. Twigg (Eds.), *Russia's Torn Safety Nets: Health and Social Welfare During the Transition* (pp. 83–99). New York: Palgrave Macmillan.

Temkina, A. (2019). 'Childbirth is not a car rental': Mothers and obstetricians negotiating consumer service in Russian commercial maternity care. *Critical Public Health*, 30(5), 521–532. http://doi.org/10.1080/09581596.2019.1626004.

Temkina, A., Litvina, D., & Novkunskaya, A. (2021). Emotional styles in Russian maternity hospitals: Juggling between khamstvo and smiling. *Emotions and Society*, 3(1), 95–113.

Temkina, A., & Rivkin-Fish, M. (2020). Creating healthcare consumers: The negotiation of un/official payments, power and trust in Russian maternity care. *Social Theory & Health*, 18(4), 340–357. http://doi.org/10.1057/s41285-019-00110-3.

Thornton, P. H., Ocasio, W., & Lounsbury, M. (2015). The institutional logics perspective. In R. A. Scott & S. M. Kosslyn (Eds.), *Emerging Trends in the Social and Behavioral Sciences*. Hoboken, NJ: John Wiley & Sons.

Timmermans, S., & Oh, H. (2010). The continued social transformation of the medical profession. *Journal of Health and Social Behavior*, 51(1), S94–S106.
Ward, K., & England, K. (2007). Introduction: Reading neoliberalization. In K. England & K. Ward (Eds.), *Neoliberalization* (pp. 1–22). Hoboken, NJ: Blackwell.
Witz, A. (2013). *Professions and Patriarchy*. Abingdon, Oxon: Routledge.
Zilber, T. B. (2016). How institutional logics matter: A bottom-up exploration. In J. Gehman, M. Lounsbury, & R. Greenwood (Eds.), *How Institutions Matter! Research in the Sociology of Organizations* (pp. 137–155). Bingley: Emerald Group Publishing Limited.

Chapter 2

"Sociologists in white"

Methodological reflections on fieldwork in maternity care

This chapter addresses the epistemological, methodological and ethical principles of our ethnographic research conducted in the biomedical field. "Sociologists in white" is an allusion to the classic book *Boys in White* (Becker et al., 1961), which explores how "boys" – medical students (at that time, predominantly male) – were becoming physicians in interactions during education. By using the category "sociologists in white," we index this study – but we center here our own professional/social performance in interactions in the empirical field. We wore medical white coats during most of our ethnographic sessions in the maternity hospital and continually reflected on how we understood our positions and identities in this field and how other participants identified us. Our empirical research is based predominantly on ethnography; thus, we open this chapter with a short description of our main methods and field sites (for detailed description of data, see Appendices 1–8). Then we provide a methodological reflection on our sociological positioning in the maternity hospital and focus on the changes that both participants and researchers undergo during their interactions.

Studying interactions in the maternity hospital: methods, field sites and data

Our interest in social studies of maternity care began several years ago and was to some extent unique for Russian academia (with exception of Rivkin-Fish, 2005). Since then, various topics related to gender and feminist studies – such as family, parenthood, sexuality, and reproduction – have been explored by many post-Soviet social scientists (including ourselves); these studies preceded and to a certain extent predefined our current research topic and our methodological positioning. While studying gender and health, we began to focus on the structural and interactional dimensions of medical settings (maternity care in particular) from a critical feminist standpoint. An integral element of these studies has been a constant process of reflection on our interactions with our research participants and on our influence on maternity care institutions and their influence on our professional identities.

DOI: 10.4324/9781003139539-2

The primary site of the research described in this book is a highly technologically developed and well-equipped maternity hospital (the Hospital) in a large Russian city. We base our analysis on ethnographic research conducted in the Hospital in 2019–2020[1] and verify it with the data that we gathered in the same and other sites during 2015–2018.

The Hospital is a state hospital of the (highest) Level 3; it provides the full spectrum of perinatal care for women and infants – from gynecology and assisted reproductive technologies to surgery and rehabilitation. Its practitioners deal with the most complicated cases of pregnancies, births and congenital disorders. The mandatory health insurance (which is obligatory and free for citizens) fully covers the cost of treatment for women and newborns, who are directed to the Hospital due to clinical indications; others must pay for its services. Conducting our research in this empirical site gave us the possibility to observe the whole complex of interactions between patients, maternity care providers and hospital administration, both within and between departments.

Our research strategy was to conduct observations in the Hospital once a week during day (and sometimes night) shifts (7.5 hours per session on average) in different departments. The idea was to follow every possible step of patients' trajectories – from reception and the emergency room to the delivery room, operating room and intensive therapy unit. Our research team was present at the Hospital on the same days, but at differing time intervals and sites. Anna and Daria were conducting ethnographic research sequentially on one department after another; while Anastasia was conducting observations of the daily routine of a chief midwife – her interactions, management and paperwork as she moved among different hospital settings. By using this strategy, we could systematically compare, clarify and triangulate our findings. Our goal was to study both interactions and general rules of organizational arrangements.

We were constantly typing field notes into our smartphones; this regime of (dis)engagement was more acceptable and common than traditional anthropological handwriting. During our fieldwork, we conducted multiple in-depth interviews and had endless situational conversations with physicians (obstetricians, neonatologists, anesthesiologists, surgeons, etc.), nurses, midwives, residents, administrators, cleaners, psychologists, and (rarely) childbearing women. We also accompanied representatives of top administration (chief physician, directors of Hospital scientific institutions, heads of departments) during their shifts, observing their routine work dealing with coordination, clinical problems, emotions and conflict resolutions. Our key gatekeeper was the director of one of the Hospital's scientific institutions (called "Director of the Hospital" for short), who would guide us into every department, introduce us to the head of that department and then leave us there on our own. Therefore, despite this top-down entry to the field, we were routinely negotiating and renegotiating our positions and explaining our professional positions and aims.

Our particular interest in this field site had emerged earlier, in 2018, when the director of the Hospital occasionally came to public lectures in which we presented the results of previous research on childbearing women and maternity care (2015–2017) (see Appendices 7–8). The director expressed interest in our studies, particularly in the ones that explained the increasing number of complaints from patients and neoliberal effects on medical professions, and agreed to become a key gatekeeper for further fieldwork. We began the study described in this book in 2018 as a series of 19 in-depth interviews with staff members and 8 patients of the Hospital (Appendix 4). In 2019, we implemented more intensive ethnographic work, which consisted of 33 observational sessions (249 hours of observation) (Appendix 3). And, finally, in 2020 we conducted 15 in-depth interviews with women who had received maternity and child services in the Hospital within the last 3 years (Appendix 2).

In this book we also refer to other sources of data from maternity care-related projects that we conducted in 2015–2017 and 2020–2021 in different locations. Our methodological reasoning for including these datasets in the current analysis is not only to broaden the scope of topics (which varied in every project) but also to verify our findings and to provide more anonymity to our participants. Herein we refer to such sources of data as interviews with childbearing women (Appendices 2, 4, 7, 8) and maternity care providers (midwives, obstetricians, etc.) (Appendices 1, 4), and analysis of media texts (Appendices 5, 6). These datasets contain information on various topics, including sensitive ones such as informal payments or abuse in delivery. In addition, we have been routinely monitoring professional medical discourses, attending medical conferences within and outside our main site, and screening relevant regulatory documents (decrees, State orders, official letters).

In every project, we conducted our research under the following ethical principles. We obtained informed consent (written or verbal and audio-recorded) from our interlocutors for their participation in the study, described to them the objectives of the study and our professional status (who we were and what we were doing) and explained the terms and conditions of using the data we gathered. When publicly presenting results in papers or publications, we provide anonymity for all our interlocutors and protect the confidentiality of the information. We also protect research data from unauthorized access and prevent the dissemination of personal facts that could potentially de-anonymize research participants.

The project "Patient-centered care in Russian healthcare: organizational challenges and professionals' opportunities," which is the key source of data for this book, was approved by two ethical committees. The first one is sociological and is located in the St Petersburg Association of Sociologists (SPAS); the other one is medical and is located at our fieldwork site. The practice of obtaining ethical permission for sociological study in Russia is still innovative and rare. In the next sections of this chapter, we explain the principles of our critical and feminist methodology and positioning as a process of negotiation and describe how we "became sociologists" in this field.

Becoming "sociologists in white": applying feminist methodology to the medical field

Ethnographic studies related to health and medicine (and to maternity care in particular) frequently take critical positions and integrate reflections on the processes of entering and working in the field (Van Hollen, 2003; Berry, 2010). Scholars argue that there is a huge potential for collaboration between the researcher and medical professionals and for integration of ethnography into medicine (Long et al., 2008). At the same time, entering the medical field is not an easy task anywhere, and in Russia this task appears to be even more challenging due to the vague ethical and legal principles of regulation of sociological research (as mentioned earlier), to low trust of "outsiders" among maternity care providers and to the unclear status of sociologists in highly hierarchical and bureaucratized medical institutions.

Outsiders in the Hospital are considered inappropriate and suspicious, and their access is limited, despite the fact that the Hospital has a lot of different inhabitants, apart from patients, their visitors, physicians, midwives and nurses. Residents, students, technical and construction workers, registrars, lawyers, psychologists, clinical researchers, visiting physicians, etc. are also part of the work and life of the facility. Nevertheless, in the Hospital (as in any other medical institution), the roles and hierarchies are clearly defined and fixed in regulatory documents, and their execution is strictly controlled – and we did not fall into any of the prescribed roles/positions. Therefore, we had to search, create and re-create not only our professional roles but also foothold for them, as such roles did not previously exist in the Hospital.

We consider our position as problematic in this field, and following the arguments of feminist methodology, we question the "neutrality" of the researcher's position and understand it as performative. We studied intrahospital communications, but we also were participants in those communications. Therefore, we continually had to clarify our professional tasks and standpoint to our interlocutors, who frequently requested this information. Methodological reflections on the process of knowledge production and positioning of the researcher in the field became important parts of our research. Nevertheless, although we never fully became "insiders," we obtained our own position and started to be considered a *svoi* ("ours"). This is a very important category of belonging to some social circle in Russia – the opposite to "outsiders." As our positioning within the Hospital was acquiring some certainty, we obtained a corresponding level of trust.

We began this project without a clear research focus or hypothesis, but we did have a general goal – to study communications within and among different departments. We were particularly attentive to the problems and failures emerging in these communications. Our understanding of communication became more complex as we deepened our knowledge while moving from one department to another, trying to understand the logics of its working interactions, institutional continuities and discontinuities. We sought to analyze the relationships between the departments, the nonlinear logistics of providing care for women and newborns in the Hospital, gaps and controversies in official regulations, and power imbalances that resulted in many informal practices that, as we discovered over time, actually set the communication patterns inside the facility.

We followed the basic principles of institutional ethnography (Smith, 2005), which is sensitive to the ruling (power) relations and positioning (standpoint) of the scholars. Institutional ethnography takes into consideration both local practices and external regulatory frames (e.g., texts) and enables researchers to uncover not only the underlying, yet ruling, relations, but also the lived experiences of real people. Beyond this, institutional ethnographers try to reorganize knowledge about "the social" so that people can use this knowledge to expand their understanding of the "local actualities" of their lives – hence, research results should be available and applicable, like a map (Smith, 2005, p. 29). Institutional ethnography starts with the researchers' standpoints within institutional contexts (ibid., p. 33). Seeing the world as problematic does not mean uncritically accepting people's interpretations and judgments. The "problematic" is something to be discovered, not the question that is concluded in the answer (Smith, 2005, p. 40). Although the people who inhabit this Hospital obviously have greater and deeper background knowledge about its inner rules, they unusually cannot "see the forest through the trees"; thus, it is sociologists who try to see the whole picture and to identify the places of different actors in the system of hierarchies and ruling relations.

During our research, we sought to explore the tensions and conflicts existing and emerging in the medical setting and among different actors; we were attentive to how people positioned themselves in the Hospital in general, in relation to each other and to us as outsiders. In this sense, we were *engaged into* these relations, and, as critical researchers, we wanted to understand these complicated relationships and hierarchies, of which we ourselves formed a temporary part. During our research, we tried to act neutrally, as we did not personally share the positionality of any our interlocutors – even when they asked or expected us to act as conflict arbitrators. We did pay attention to emotions, both our own and those of our participants, as they carry strong interpretive potential and can help to understand the underlying and often otherwise invisible nature of staff, patient and researcher communications.

The guiding principles of our study derive from feminist epistemology and methodology (Reinharz, 1993; Zdravomyslova & Temkina, 2014) and include the ethics of care, collaboration between researchers and participants, recognition of personal experiences and the desire to empower the participants with new knowledge that could enhance their understandings of themselves, their interlocutors and the context in which they are situated. Thus, empirical research requires a certain type of cognizant researcher who is oriented toward the creation of egalitarian relationships, toward reducing the distance between researcher and research participant and toward implementing emotional labor and care. Feminist ethics are characterized by sensitivity to power relations, problematizing the exploitation of interlocutors as objects of cognition, and striving for egalitarian dialogue. Therefore, reflexivity – and the researchers themselves – become important instruments in the process of knowledge production. However, in actual practice, these "ideal" principles are problematic in and of themselves, as we will show.

The sociologist in the medical field is an obscure figure for its inhabitants – her legal, professional, political and bodily conditions are under constant investigation. Who is this person? Can she be trusted? Formally, we had become "medical sociologists" as soon as we entered the Hospital and began observations, yet our entrance into the field was never fully completed, as our positions were never fixed nor clearly determined for all of our interlocutors. Our positions were always fluid: we were constantly examined and identified in various ways. We felt keenly the volatility of the researcher's role and of her positionality.

Conventionally, the progressive transition from one position to another is discussed as a path from "outsider" to "insider" and sometimes to "participant" (Flick, 2006; Hammersley & Atkinson, 2019). We show that none of these positions were ever fully acquired in our case. The researcher in the field may not be allowed to participate in the most important activities in the field and therefore become an insider; or she may be partially involved in them; or may be a full member of the studied group (Adler & Adler, 1987). In the latter case, the researcher shares the values and identities of the field as insider. We argue that a clear separation of researchers from participants has more analytical than practical implications; in practice researchers may find themselves in situations of role conflict or ambiguity (Adler & Adler, 1987).

The extreme positions of insider and outsider are analytically distinctive, but they are not necessarily opposed: the researcher may not obtain any of them – for example, when exploring the grief experienced due to the death of loved ones in disasters (see Breen, 2007); the research may include both perspectives when co-researchers have different experiences (see, e.g., Dwyer & Buckle, 2009 on perinatal loss); the researcher may constantly switch from one position to another (see, e.g., Paechter, 2013 on using a pseudonym as a website participant and a real name as a researcher of online spaces for the divorced); or the researchers may position themselves as "critical friends" (Swaffield & MacBeath, 2005; Fletcher, 2019).

The researcher can be completely outside, or somewhere in-between, the insider-outsider binary; from a feminist perspective, the boundaries between the researcher and the researched are permeable. A dialectical approach is more suitable to understanding the insider-outsider dilemma – the hyphen indexes that ambivalent space "in-between" (Breen, 2007; Humphrey, 2007; Dwyer & Buckle, 2009; Kerstetter, 2012; Paechter, 2013; Fletcher, 2019). We believe that the insider-outsider continuum provides necessary, but not sufficient, grounds for understanding the researcher's position in the field.

As previously noted, we had to explain to our Hospital interlocutors *ad infinitum* who we were and what we were doing there, and to work to create trust. During our fieldwork, we were constantly maneuvering in our interactions with these interlocutors and shifting in their perceptions from one role to another (Harrington, 2003). We argue that the researcher never truly becomes an insider – she can at any time lose her status, her access to the field, and the trust she has worked so hard to build, become an outsider, and has to start all over again. Moreover, especially in institutional settings, she may not want to become an insider or have no such option.

During our research, our position as knowers constantly shifted, in Haraway's terms (1988), from a position of knowledge production from "nowhere" (when we tried to be as invisible as possible, such as in operating rooms or intensive care units) to "somewhere" (when participants appealed to us as arbiters or referred to our research results to argue for their own positions and theories). As we shifted among multiple positions, we constantly constructed and performed ourselves as sociologists. Participants did not take our positions for granted, and we ourselves were never confident in our roles in this field. We learned that the process of performing ourselves and our interactions becomes research data itself and was key to the interpretation of our whole dataset.

To deepen this methodological reflection, we need to clarify some peculiarities of State-funded medical facilities in Russia. These are closed, hierarchical and overregulated communities, where health and maternity care providers are often in vulnerable positions compared to their Western counterparts (Litvina et al., 2019), emotionally overwhelmed (especially when dealing with existential issues of life and death) and extremely suspicious of unfamiliar visitors (like us). Access to hospitals for non-inhabitants is usually restricted. Even when researchers have professional skills, a perfect gatekeeper, a good team and strong ethical principles, still, after initial entry, they have to repeatedly explain and confirm their position. Yet no matter how much and how often we explained our professional status, we still faced multiple cases of misidentification.

Analytically, we have identified several situations of interactions in which the position of the sociologist in the field was explicitly problematized, which we describe in the following sections: (1) identification (What is a sociologist?); (2) examination (What do they know? What do they want? Which side they are on?); (3) "doing sociologists" in interaction (How to treat them? What are the rules for them?); (4) creating trust (Is it possible to trust them? To what extent?). As we dealt with these dimensions, we were changing the field we were working in and that field was changing us.

Identifying the sociologist

We always started every new episode of communication in a new department with a short presentation of ourselves, our ethnographic plans, and our ethical principles. Sometimes we had to do this very briefly and quickly, as the care providers were extremely busy. Some of them (mostly those in administrative positions) remembered us from our presentation at the Hospital's medical conference, but usually during the first steps in communication we were identified as psychologists, social workers, conflict managers, journalists, residents, visitors, or even as representatives of controlling bodies. For most of our interlocutors, it was unclear from the very beginning who and what sociologists are and what they can do in a medical facility; thus, practitioners sought to fit us into a category that they already understood.

During one of our ethnographic sessions, Anastasia followed the chief midwife and the hospital's epidemiologist, who were inspecting the departments on the eve of the visit of representatives from two major outside controlling bodies – Roszdravnadzor and Rospotrebnadzor (for more details see Chapter 3). They were inspecting departments and wards for meeting sanitary norms and various other formal requirements. The chief midwife introduced Anastasia: "This is a sociologist," and the epidemiologist nodded contentedly, saying: "Oh, I also had conflict management classes at the university!" (field notes), misidentifying sociologists as conflict specialists. During the inspection, other participants behaved as if the sociologist was an epidemiologist assistant and did not problematize her presence, as a large number of local and external inspections is routine in medical institutions. Sociology, epidemiology and conflict management seemed to be synonymous in this situation – as in the eyes of our interlocutors, the researcher was particularly interested in inspection and investigation of conflicts and "rules," despite her attempt to explicitly announce her professional status.

Another set of field notes illustrates a situation in which our professional work (taking notes, asking questions) was interpreted in a very ambivalent way, with the sociologist seen as a possible "spy" and "examined" for sincerity and trust:

> *15.00 [Olga] (the chief nurse of department 1) enters the room and asks whether [Irina Nikolaevna] (the chief physician) is present and starts talking with [Natalia] (head of department 2). [Natalia] sees me and smiles (her look tells me that she sees me as a spy).*

Olga: I want a vacation!
Natalia: Get sick then!
Olga: I don't want to get sick!
Natalia: Then fake it.
Olga: I don't want to fake it either.
[Natalia] looks at me and laughs: "Hey, Asya keeps writing there! She will spread it around later!"

I also laugh, but since then I keep thinking what my actions look like from outside and try to look at my phone less often (field notes).

Anastasia (Asya) realized that she was being labeled as a spy (ironically, but still . . .) who was collecting information about informal negotiations (discussion of participants about possibly faking sickness to have some days off) in order to "report" this to the head (for a similar story, see Wind, 2008). Anastasia as sociologist was placed in the local hierarchy of subordination and information transfer, where even a "neutral" academic position is considered problematic.

Examining/testing the sociologist

Even when we were recognized as researchers, that recognition did not lead directly to an understanding of our purposes. Our professionalism was tested in various situations. The following field note episode by Daria Livina (DL) illustrates this situation of strict examination:

At some point a woman (Diana) approaches us. I immediately identify her as a nurse – not sure why. She starts the communication quite abruptly and asks who we are and where do we come from. I explain that we are sociologists. "Are you part of the staff?" I explain that we are not and that we have a collaborative project and our presence here is authorized by the head of the department and by administration.

Diana: What is the aim of the study? Subject and object? Are you students? – she nods at me and Anna Temkina.
Anna: I am a professor!
Diana: Sorry [doesn't sound like she is sorry at all].

Then [Diana] asks questions about our university, our experience, our knowledge about the situation abroad. At the moment when she asked if we were students, I started to think that this is a kind of verification/provocation (because it is hard to confuse Anna with a student). According to the reaction of another nurse who is standing by Diana, I understand that it is not a stalemate situation – the nurse is smiling.

But I realize that I have to speak cautiously, so that the field (or part of it) wouldn't collapse. Anna joins our conversation and starts explaining our project. Diana says that any project has object and subject – what are they? I feel like the conversation strikes up (at least in some direction) and say that I guess I don't know her name. She introduces herself [DL: says only the first name, which is quite informal]. I ask what is her position. She says she is the chief nurse of this department. That's when we switch into dialogue mode (still led by her). Then it gets better.

(field notes)

We had to prove that we are "real sociologists" – according to the ideas of our interlocutor about the nature of research work, which we had to fit. Since we were outsider sociologists (there are no local ones in the Hospital), she felt that she had to test not only our knowledge but also our loyalty, and – most important – our status and identity. (How would we react if she deliberately lowered our status? How we would demonstrate our professionalism?) Adjusting to this communication style (which was more or less common to most of our interlocutors) required emotional labor and self-assurance in our identity as "sociologists in white" (which, again, was continually in the making). Tensions could arise when we couldn't adjust quickly – usually due to the complexity of informal rules, symbols and contexts which we were unfamiliar with (and tried to explore). To fit in as insiders, all inhabitants of the medical field must learn the unwritten rules of communication, as we will explain later, and if some outsiders (e.g. sociologists, patients, new staff members) do not understand such rules and do not obey them, this leads to problems in communication.

"Doing sociologists" in interaction

We were constantly in the process of "doing sociologists," which is analogous to "doing gender," where "gender [is] a kind of a doing, an incessant activity performed . . . an improvisation within a scene of constraint. Moreover, one does not 'do' gender alone. One is always 'doing' with or for another" (Butler, 2004, p. 3). Our Hospital interlocutors always treated us differently, trying to find an appropriate form of communication with us and to discipline our bodies in their own ways, as in this field note from Daria Litvina's diary:

A nurse Ira leads us (me and Anna Temkina) to the sanitary room. She gives us full instruction on how to dress properly. She gives us dispensable covers and says that we must put on the cap and the shoe covers when we step on the yellow floor in the operational zone. On the inside I am surprised – I didn't expect that we will go to the operation room. Ira offers us to put our belongings into her locker and says that we can

> *leave our stuff here – nobody will take it, there is no thieving here. . . . When she drops the packages from our covers into the trash, she by the way reminds us not to forget about the yellow and white buckets (they are for different sorts of trash). I ask her to remind us about the buckets. I think that at this moment she understands that something is wrong because she asks who we are. We say that we are sociologists. She asks why are we here and what do we want. I tell her about our study of the communications in the hospital. She doesn't understand what type of communication I am talking about. I say, about the one between the physician and the patient. Ira says that nowadays patients are so impudent that they record them on the phone . . .*
>
> *After some time comes the head of the department. He takes our caps and shoe covers and says we won't need them. Then we go to the operation room. I feel like it is inconvenient to take notes – don't know why, but I do not take the phone out. We approach the operation room and step on that yellow floor right in front of the entrance to it. I kind of worry about that, because we had to be in shoe covers at that point. The operation is in process and I can feel the specific smell – like the one during the laser epilation (or maybe it only seems alike to me). In the operation room there are several people who are in the same dispensable covers as we are. One of them (anesthesiologist) is questioningly looking at us and the head of the department is waving his hand – nothing, don't get distracted. The surgeons are focused on the operation. We get out of there quite quickly.*
>
> *(field notes)*

Bodily regulations depend on professional positions and places in the Hospital's hierarchy. If we were (interpreted as) medical practitioners (in this situation we were probably identified by a nurse as a professor and her resident), we would have to follow sanitary norms; however, these norms are apparently not obligatory for sociologists. Being a sociologist in medical settings also means frequently breaking the rules – because the ones for sociologists are not yet designed. If we were maternity care providers, we would have had to wear all protective equipment, but when we were identified as sociologists, this became unnecessary. Hierarchy also matters: the nurse insisted we should be equipped; the chief of the department did not. Our feelings were ambivalent; we were not clear about what rules we should follow and how we should behave. Both of us (Anna and Daria) felt that in the operating room, we could not take notes, as we were not quite sociologists in that place, nor were we maternity care providers. At such times, we often felt that we existed in some interdimensional realm where nothing was transparent and everything was opaque. We continuously sought to comprehend how we could produce ourselves when we were interpreted as assistants, residents, obstetricians, inspectors, epidemiologists, spies, etc. Our participants were intensively involved in the process of producing us as sociologists – they dressed or undressed us, showed us the places where we could and could not be and explained to us their understandings of what a sociologist is, which rarely matched our own.

In our attempts to answer the questions "who are you?" and "what is your position in this setting?" we came to the simple formulaic statement that we were "sociologists in a medical facility" – a self-sufficient position. But in order to fit this simple formula, it was not enough to just present ourselves as scholars. We needed to create not only our position but also our corporeal and emotional relevance to it. At the beginning of our fieldwork, we did not wear white coats (and nobody demanded that we do so), as we didn't understand our position and didn't want to be misidentified as physicians. But after approximately one month of intensive work, we finally put on white coats, in order to appear as professionals who belonged in the Hospital, who dressed not like visitors but like actual staff members, as the white coat symbolizes a professional position in a hospital. Given that there is a variety of practitioners within the hospital who wear white coats, in donning them, we created ourselves as another set of professionals. This did not feel like cultural appropriation. We didn't pretend to occupy someone else's position, but received our own in multiple interactions and became "sociologists in white coats" – from this standpoint, we further continued to reproduce our professional identities and positions.

Over time, from some of our participants' perspectives, we went from being "some sociologists" to "our sociologists." Our hard work on establishing trust began to pay off and our research began to flow more smoothly as we moved into becoming "our sociologists" – but, as we have noted earlier, this is not the same as an insider position. In an ongoing process of negotiations and interactions, we (together with participants) created the position of "a sociologist in a hospital," which had never existed there before – the one which is neither fully inside or outside the field. Our white coats did symbolically mark our belonging to the field, but our position was still situationally created in every interaction. Sociologists had not previously existed here – at the beginning, we were either invisible or suspicious figures, but in the process of interaction, our positionality mutated through a continuous and never-ending process of creation. In contexts of medical organizations, a sociologist is positioned not only in terms of belonging to the field but also in the degree of foreignness to its rules and cultures. The creation of this position is influenced not only by how we want to identify ourselves within the field but also how we are identified. This took the shape of a constant movement backward and forward in the insider/outsider dichotomy. We argue that having a clear standpoint and *caring* about our interlocutors and their patients are important for obtaining trust.

Creating trust in interactions

As a result, we not only repetitively articulated our positions within the investigated field but also ultimately managed to establish relationships that both presupposed and produced trust. Despite our relatively successful communications with our participants, the fear that we would lose trust persisted. Trust could exist in one moment but could be lost in another. Sometimes it emerged in unpredictable and unplanned situations, including the most dramatic ones, when we felt an emotional overlap with our interlocutors, a feeling that we were wanted as people who could share the moment:

> *Irina Nikolaevna and Elena Vladimirovna are sitting in the room. Irina says that they are discussing the meaning of everything, the meaning of profession. In front of them lies a medical file approximately four centimeters thick. This night another woman died.*
>
> ***Irina:*** *Every case like that is a scar (about the death). Every time when you go to autopsy, you never fully know whether something was missed. This time there was (a substantial reason), nobody is guilty. But each of 20 people who were present felt themselves sort of guilty. Right, Ekaterina?*
> ***Elena:*** *Absolutely.*
> ***Irina:*** *The head of the department is a very advanced woman. She wrote a message that she will probably have to quit (her job here). She says that during the examination it was not pronounced, but she feels like that. . . . Of course, she wouldn't quit. But every time – on the verge.*
>
> *Irina and Elena thank us (me and Anna) for listening – they say that it makes it easier for them. Denis Sergeevich said the same today after the interview. I hope it is so (field note).*

As a result of this situational conversation related to the death of a childbearing woman who had been hospitalized with multiple complications, we came to comprehend one more dimension of our positionality. Participants were grateful to us for listening, for understanding and accepting their position (we were *somewhere*) and for our empathetic comprehension of the suffering of maternity care providers, and not just the suffering of the relatives of the deceased. This brings us back to the question of holding a position in which we could not just show up and collect data from nowhere – we had to get involved, talk, care, position ourselves and build ourselves into local relationships and structures, both from somewhere (the inside) and from nowhere (the outside).

We discovered that this is how an unofficial, yet legitimate, position of a sociologist emerges in the medical setting – not spelled out anywhere, but obviously existing. We had been changing ourselves because we found ourselves in situations that we did not expect to see and feel, and this was a mutual process. Interaction between scholars and research participants/interlocutors is a bilateral process that reveals new knowledge both for the researcher and for the interviewee as the researcher guides the latter through sequential reflection (Patton, 1990). Ethnographic research cannot be limited to "getting the needed data" – it must be acknowledged as having the potential to change both the researcher and her field. Moreover, beyond some concerns about potential biases, many researchers see huge analytical potential in the emotional responses that we see, feel or produce in the field: "The greatest source of analytic value occurs during what we call the emotional overlap, or those moments during fieldwork when the emotions of both the informant and the ethnographer are shared" (Feldman & Mandache, 2019, p. 229). Whenever we ignore or exclude those moments from analysis as "biases," we impoverish our dataset and ourselves.

Conclusion: creating our standpoint

The process of ethnographic work in medical settings includes not only reflection on one's position but also constant (re)production of this position. Our standpoint is not something we recognize, but something we create or, more precisely, start to recognize in the moment when we have to create it. We partially change the field even if we try to remain neutral-invisible-imperceptible (to be "nowhere"), as participants in our study often want to clarify our positions and perceive *us* as interlocutors (place us "somewhere"). Some traces of our presence and configurations of interactions that we have created remain in the field even after we exit it, both in the hearts and minds of our participants and via publication of our research results. These become publicly available and maternity care providers refer to them, using them as the "map" we intended them to be, and sometimes building more sustainable relationships with us over time. When we change the field and the field changes us, we cannot tell ourselves that we are just "collecting data" anymore. Because – both physically and emotionally – we have already become participants, we are insiders, we are somewhere – and then with the next project or person, we start as outsiders all over again. Our fieldwork experiences have taught us that in complicated field settings, switching among different roles can be beneficial. Our differential placements can make our vision of our field stereoscopic, even as we adhere to our standpoint and to our principle of emotional caring – which ultimately are what allows us to obtain deep and trustworthy narratives and varied field experiences.

Note

1 The research was conducted with the support of the Russian Science Foundation (grant N 19-78-10128). It was a part of a project called "Patient-centered care in Russian healthcare: organizational challenges and professionals' opportunities" conducted at the European University at Saint Petersburg. We express our gratitude to the head of the project, Ekaterina Borozdina, for supporting our research.

References

Adler, P., & Adler, P. (1987). *Membership Roles in Field Research*. Newbury Park, CA: Sage.

Becker, H. S., Geer, B., Hughes, E. C., & Strauss, A. L. (1961). *Boys in White: Student Culture in Medical School*. Chicago: The University of Chicago Press.

Berry, N. (2010). *Unsafe Motherhood: Mayan Maternal Mortality and Subjectivity in Post-War Guatemala*. New York and Oxford: Berghahn Books.

Breen, L. (2007). The researcher 'in the middle': Negotiating the insider/outsider dichotomy. *The Australian Community Psychologist*, 19(1), 163–174.

Butler, J. (2004). *Undoing Gender*. New York and London: Routledge.

Dwyer, S. C., & Buckle, J. L. (2009). The space between: On being an insider-outsider in qualitative research. *International Journal of Qualitative Methods*, 8(1), 54–63.

Feldman, L. R., & Mandache, L.-A. (2019). Emotional overlap and the analytic potential of emotions in anthropology. *Ethnography*, 20(2), 227–244.

Fletcher, A. (2019). An invited outsider or an enriched insider? Challenging contextual knowledge as a critical friend researcher. In S. Plowright, M. Green, & N. F. Johnson (Eds.), *Educational Researchers and the Regional University: Agents of Regional-global Transformation* (pp. 75–92). Singapore: Springer.

Flick, U. (2006). *An Introduction to Qualitative Research*. London: Sage Publications.

Hammersley, M., & Atkinson, P. (2019). *Ethnography: Principles in Practice* (4th ed.). London and New York: Routledge.

Haraway, D. (1988). Situated knowledges: The science question in feminism and the privilege of partial perspective. *Feminist Studies*, 14(3), 575–599.

Harrington, B. (2003). The social psychology of access in ethnographic research. *Journal of Contemporary Ethnography*, 32(5), 592–625.

Humphrey, C. (2007). Insider-outsider: Activating the hyphen. *Action Research*, 5(1), 11–26.

Kerstetter, K. (2012). Insider, outsider, or somewhere between: The impact of researchers' identities on the community-based research process. *Journal of Rural Social Sciences*, 27(2), 99–117.

Litvina, D., Novkunskaya, A., & Temkina, A. (2019). Multiple vulnerabilities in medical settings: Invisible suffering of doctors. *Societies*, 10(1), 5. https://doi.org/10.3390/soc10010005.

Long, D., Hunter, C., & Van der Geest, S. (2008). When the field is a ward or a clinic: Hospital ethnography. *Anthropology & Medicine*, 15(2), 71–78.

Paechter, C. (2013). Researching sensitive issues online: Implications of a hybrid insider/outsider position in a retrospective ethnographic study. *Qualitative Research*, 13(1), 71–86.
Patton, M. Q. (1990). *Qualitative Evaluation and Research Methods* (2nd ed.). Newbury Park: Sage Publications.
Reinharz, S. (1993). Neglected voices and excessive demand in feminist research. *Qualitative Sociology*, 16(1), 69–76.
Rivkin-Fish, M. (2005). *Women's Health in Post-Soviet Russia: The Politics of Intervention.* Bloomington and Indianapolis: Indiana University Press.
Smith, D. E. (2005). *Institutional Ethnography: A Sociology for People.* Lanham: AltaMira Press.
Swaffield, S., & MacBeath, J. (2005). School self-evaluation and the role of a critical friend. *Cambridge Journal of Education*, 35(2), 239–252.
Van Hollen, C. (2003). *Birth on the Threshold: Childbirth and Modernity in South India.* Berkeley, Los Angeles, and London: University of California Press.
Wind, G. (2008). Negotiated interactive observation: Doing fieldwork in hospital settings. *Anthropology & Medicine*, 15(2), 79–89.
Zdravomyslova, E., & Temkina, A. (2014). Feminist reflections on fieldwork [Feministskie refleksii o polevom issledovanii]. *Laboratorium*, 6(1), 84–112 (In Russian).

Chapter 3

Maternity care in Russia

The Soviet legacy and post-Soviet reforms

In spite of the universal, free-of-charge access to maternity care inherited from the Soviet healthcare system, childbearing women in Russia are often not able to get the services they want, and maternity care providers often cannot meet women's expectations and needs. In this chapter, we address the key preconditions of this state of affairs. We ask and answer the questions of how the organization of maternity care and its ongoing reformations have affected the positions of women and providers, and their encounters. We describe the historical, structural and ideological backgrounds of Russian maternity care, with particular attention to the legacy of Soviet state paternalism and to the current marketization in the course of neoliberal reforms.

The Russian public system of maternity care provides universal medical help for women and newborns during preconception, pregnancy, labor and the postpartum period. The standard route of a pregnant woman includes the monitoring of pregnancy in State-funded outpatient facilities called "women's consultations" (*zhenskaya consultatsia*), and giving birth in maternity hospitals (*rodil'niye doma*) (as we will describe at the end of this chapter). This State-funded maternity care is "free" for citizens – it is covered by mandatory health insurance (MHI). The recent commercialization of care partially changed the healthcare landscape; however, private maternity units are rare and are located only in large cities. Many state-funded facilities also provide additional commercial services (along with the free basic services) that offer more comfort and better services for women (Temkina, 2016).

In general, childbirth is highly medicalized in Russia: childbirth assistance is legal only in medical facilities, and every childbirth must be attended by (at least) an obstetrician, midwife and neonatologist.[1] Midwives alone cannot monitor pregnancies and assist with delivery (Ministry of Health, 2012). Attending homebirth is prohibited for health providers and can lead to legal problems for all participants in case of complications. Nevertheless, some parents choose home or "alternative" childbirth, and some birth attendants support them in actualizing that choice (Borozdina, 2014; Novkunskaya, 2014; Ozhiganova, 2019).

Maternity care is highly centralized in Russia; it is directly governed and rigidly controlled by various State bodies and mandatory insurance companies.

DOI: 10.4324/9781003139539-3

Nowadays, key among these are the Ministry of Health; the Mandatory Health Insurance federal and regional funds; the Russian Federal Service for Surveillance on Consumer Rights Protection and Human Wellbeing *(Rospotrebnadzor)*; the Federal Service for Surveillance in Healthcare (*Roszdravnadzor*); and federal and regional authorities. In cases of legal proceedings, the Investigating Committee (*Sledstvenniy Komitet*) comes into play. These key decision-makers in this field impose a top-down approach to healthcare management, and there are multiple references in our empirical data to these bodies, their demands and numerous inspections; sometimes they are jointly referred to as "the System." The rules that regulate and coordinate this system often contradict each other and are unclear and non-transparent, as we will show.

The following analysis of the macro-structural level of maternity care acknowledges the State's extensive control and the subordinated position of both maternity care providers (mostly state employees) and childbearing women in Russia. We analyze contemporary Russian maternity care as a "*hybrid*" that has been shaped in the process of post-Soviet reforms by:

(1) the legacy of the Soviet paternalistic principles of universal, centralized and medicalized healthcare;
(2) managerial/bureaucratic principles of post-Soviet state paternalism; and
(3) neoliberal marketization.

We begin this chapter by describing the Soviet healthcare principles that have significantly shaped the current institutional arrangements and the rules of Russian healthcare in general, and maternity care in particular. We then focus on the top-down approach to reforming and regulating maternity services during the post-Soviet period: the decentralization of care in the 1990s, and the pronatalist turn in the mid-2000s, followed by re-centralization and numerous reforms in the 2010s.

In the following section, we turn to the analysis of the multiple inconsistencies that are palpable at the levels of both regulatory rules and practices: lack of continuity of care in the trajectory of childbearing women across different medical facilities, and the inconsistency of the rules in maternity hospitals. We argue that as the result of the "hybridization" of different Soviet and post-Soviet rules in maternity care's organization, its participants can neither provide nor receive good care by default, but have to redefine and struggle to achieve it.

The Soviet legacy: paternalism in centralized maternity care

Paternalism used to be the dominant pattern in relations between the State and the citizens in Soviet society – and to a great extent still is, as we will demonstrate. Herein we introduce the Soviet historical background and explore how the Soviet legacy still largely shapes the current arrangement and provision of maternity care – a part of universal healthcare. We conceptualize Soviet maternity care as *paternalistic System* and explore how it affects the participants – providers and childbearing women – as well as the quality of care. Scholars argue that paternalistic practices implementing power and authority have medical and moral (normative) dimensions (Larivaara, 2010; Leykin, 2011). Paternalism in health and maternity care presupposes normative patterns of hierarchical power relationships within medical institutions. These patterns reveal themselves in disciplining top-down organizational practices and are morally proved as the legitimate "good care" of the superiors – the obstetricians who "know best" about the subordinates – childbearing women.

Paternalism reveals itself in the interactions between the State and the medical institutions and between maternity care providers and their patients within medical facilities. In the top-down style of regulation, the State (the Federal Government, the Ministry of Health, and other bodies) decides what institutional arrangements and reforms serve the common good and provide "good care" for citizens. In this system, physicians become translators of State politics in healthcare, while patients become passive recipients of care (see also Bogdanova, 2021 on the State's paternalistic care of citizens who file official complaints). On the institutional level, paternalism operates as a set of imperatives and rules that frame hierarchical positions and encounters. Hereby, patients are subordinated to providers, and providers are directly subordinated to the hospital administration and to the State's ruling bodies.

There are some prominent historical studies that trace the legacy of certain factors – such as the medicalization of childbirth and the subordination of midwifery to obstetrics – from even *pre*-revolutionary Russia (Pushkareva & Mitsyuk, 2017). However, we start our analysis in the Soviet period and focus on key characteristics. Among the main principles in Soviet healthcare, called the "Semashko model" (introduced by Nikolai Semashko, the first People's Commissar of Public Health in 1918–1930), were universal access and centralization in terms of regulation, financing and service provision (Younger, 2016, p. 1086). These included state-funded medical facilities (health workers were salaried from the State's budget) and systematic, direct top-down administrative control (Sheiman et al., 2018, p. 209).

The second principle of Soviet healthcare was its universal accessibility for all citizens across the country. Health and maternity care were provided "for free" under a "territorial" principle – people could get medical help in certain polyclinics and hospitals, which were predetermined according to their *propiska* (registered place of residence) without any choice. Some additional healthcare coverage could be provided by the organization where a citizen was employed. The territorial principle was relevant for both maternity and newborn care – women could not pick medical facilities or providers of their choice and had only one option of getting obstetric help for themselves or their babies – that help came from the nearby institution to which they were assigned. Only in the very rural areas of the country, as other scholars demonstrate, could some women still give birth at home with traditional midwives, as even "peasant" women born after the Revolution women accepted and followed many norms of the pre-Soviet village, including homebirth (Adonyeva & Olson, 2011). However, homebirth was not an option for most Soviet women and emerged in cities as an intentionally dissident (and illegal) practice only in the 1980s (Belooussova, 2002). In general, the Semashko model proved to be effective in terms of solving problems related to public health, including accessibility, disease prevention and hygiene. However, during the Soviet era (1922–1991), and especially at its end in the early 1990s, the health and maternity care systems were characterized by a deficit of modern equipment, lack of drugs and disposable items and overcrowded wards with insufficient staff (Paton, 1989, p. 45).

During the Soviet era, all health and maternity care providers were exclusively State employees, received fixed salaries from the State and reported to hospital administration and governmental bodies rather than to patients or professional organizations (Field, 1957; Rivkin-Fish, 2005; Saks, 2015). The centralization of care – presupposed by systematic, top-down obligatory instructions and down-up obligatory accountability to the State – entailed unitary rigid rules and control. Physicians were meant to strictly follow the laws, recommendations, procedures and rules. As a result, maternity care providers in Soviet hospitals lacked autonomy and personal responsibility for childbearing women (Brown, 1987). Interactions with patients were mostly depersonalized in a "conveyer-belt-like" system (Rivkin-Fish, 2005) in which women had no choices, physicians did not have enough time and none of them had sufficient resources. Providers had a high level of differentiation of tasks, as several physicians of different specializations monitored pregnancy, while others assisted with birth and the postpartum period. In other words, there was a complete lack of continuity of care. State-employed practitioners were poorly paid, politically inert and had extremely limited autonomy (Field, 1957; Saks, 2015). Public and professional voices had little or no space in this paternalistic system (Gaal & McKee, 2004, p. 171).

Paternalism revealed itself as a principle of relationships between care providers and receivers ("doctor knows best"); powerless patients had equal and free access to care, but most of them lacked personalized care and attention. (See Chapter 5 for an analysis of the abusive communicative practice of *khamstvo*, which is a trait specific to (post)Soviet paternalism.)

On the level of interactions, Soviet maternity care was embedded in a lack of privacy and supply, depersonalization, neglect and humiliation. The physical environment and the inner rules of maternity hospitals did not provide any sort of privacy for childbearing women (e.g., birth rooms were shared by many women in labor, and no personal belongings, including underwear, were allowed, due to "sanitary standards"). Mothers were separated from their newborns immediately after birth and the babies were whisked away to the newborn nurseries (immediate skin-to-skin contact was not practiced), breastfeeding was limited (it was supposed that mothers should feed newborns at certain time intervals), and no visitors were allowed (including women's partners). This was an entirely industrialized system of birth with no room in it for humanistic connections of mothers to babies nor to their care providers (see Davis-Floyd, 2018; Davis-Floyd & Cheyney, 2022). International recommendations and ideals of maternity care mostly did not penetrate the Soviet model of childbirth, which had its own paternalistic, medicalized ideals of "good care."

In an interview, Zhenya, an obstetrician aged 52, described Soviet maternity care as follows:

> *There were postnatal wards [in the mid-1990], for twelve people – the big, big ones. Naturally, these weren't wards where mothers and babies are kept together – the babies had been brought there [and then brought back to neonatal wards].*

Childbearing women usually felt uncomfortable and scared; they received very few explanations during labor and after birth and had no personal contact with birth assistants. Providers considered women to be ignorant and expected them to follow their experts' instructions and to endure pain, suffering and medical interventions. Pregnant and laboring women were supposed to be passively obedient to medical providers, as there were no alternatives and no opportunities to negotiate a more personalized approach, though with some exceptions.

Some women tried to receive better care by using informal referrals (*blat*) and unofficial out-of-pocket payments to achieve some degree of choice and to establish more personalized relationships with physicians (see also Chapter 4). They tried to find someone whom they personally knew related to maternity care whom they could trust and who would arrange their treatment and manage their births. This informal personalization used to be the only way to overcome institutional rigidity and to get more patient-oriented care. Women strove to create trusting relations with obstetricians, whom they found by mobilizing their social networks (Rivkin-Fish, 2005; Stepurko et al., 2013).

Extensive State control and insufficient finances resulted in patients' and providers' deep dissatisfaction with the quality of healthcare and the growth of unofficial horizontal practices as their coping strategies. After the Soviet collapse, healthcare institutions continued to work in the same way, yet some measures to improve care were made. In the next section, we take a closer look at the reforms that have adapted and reconfigured the Soviet legacy and also have changed the whole landscape of health and maternity care in Russia.

Post-Soviet reforms: the hybridization of maternity care

Since the collapse of the USSR in 1991, substantial political, economic and social changes gave rise to new arrangements and regulations of health and maternity care. Especially noticeable changes occurred at the beginning of the 2000s, when maternity services – still highly medicalized, extensively bureaucratized and rigidly regulated by the State – at the same time became more oriented to the market principles of care provision and control. They also became more competitive and more oriented to patients' growing consumeristic demands. This hybrid system, which combined neoliberal market principles with State paternalism, consequently led to contradictions and inconsistencies in institutional arrangements and to multiple problems in the coordination and continuity of health services within and between facilities. These inconsistencies posed new challenges both for women acquiring maternity care and the practitioners providing it. In order to explain this hybridization of regulatory logics in the field of maternity care in Russia, we refer to the post-Soviet reforms that took place during the 1990s, especially in the 2000s. In particular, we focus on effects on the quality of care ("good care") and the positions of the key actors inhabiting this field.

Reforms of the 1990s: decentralization and fragmentation of health and maternity care

The *Perestroika* period (in the late 1980s) launched a course toward "renewal" and entailed the growth of economic markets and the diminishment of centralization and central planning. During the 1990s, a changing political and economic landscape shaped particular arrangements and the regulatory frameworks of maternity care. Substantial commercialization of services occurred during this period, which was characterized by the emergence of commercial private clinics and paid-for services within "free" public medical organizations (Borozdina, 2014). Governmental management of this sphere became palpably more liberal, particularly due to decentralization: more autonomy in decision-making was given to regional authorities. Scholars identify this non-systematic process of liberalization as "chaotic privatization and decentralization of the welfare responsibilities" (Jäppinen et al., 2011, pp. 2–3). The economic liberalization of health and maternity care was implemented through targeting reforms and the introduction of a Mandatory Health Insurance model in 1993 (Younger, 2016, p. 1087). These innovations established the principles of market regulation and were intended to reduce the role of the State, thereby highlighting in retrospect its ineffective rigidity and inflexibility during the Soviet period (Twigg, 1998).

Another way to overcome the rigidity and obsolescence of the paternalistic State-led model of maternity care was internationalization, which occurred through various international programs and collaborations. With the support of the World Health Organization (WHO) and UNICEF, a new federal program of "Safe motherhood" was launched (1995–2001). It included the promotion of the Baby-friendly Hospital Initiative (which supports breastfeeding and keeping mothers and newborns together) in some maternity hospitals, and the opening of new "Centers of family planning" in various regions, which offered consultations concerning contraception and abortion prevention (Chalmers, 1997, 2022; Rivkin-Fish, 2005). Owing to the decentralized and non-consistent regulations of these initiatives and to unequal distribution of both material and social resources across regions, the transformation of maternity services was patchy.

During the 1990s, the quality and accessibility of Russian social services in general, and maternity services in particular, became uneven. Regionalization, fragmentation and non-systematic improvements generated new types of social inequality between and within regions. Innovations were not always appreciated at the federal level (Cook, 2017, p. 13), and new regional disparities in the accessibility and quality of health and maternity care services emerged (Shuvalova et al., 2015; Shishkin et al., 2017, p. 9). At the end of the 1980s, there was a large deficit in supply, and poor conditions were widespread; this situation continued and, in some cases, was even aggravated in the 1990s. Zina, a mother, age 56, describes the poor economic conditions of that period in maternity care:

> *It was the time, you know . . . The year 1990 is a special chapter in our history, right? [because the Soviet era was ending]. It is not that there was just nothing there, . . . there was nothing at all.*

Zina explains that in addition to poor conditions, there were no gloves nor sufficient supplies of other types of needed equipment in maternity hospitals – mothers had to bring everything on their own. This sharp scarcity of material resources was common in State-funded medical facilities. Due to the economic and political crises taking place at that time, the State-funded sectors suffered most of all, and some of the welfare and healthcare reforms resulted in the deterioration of service provision and of healthcare providers' working conditions.

The neoliberal reforms of the 1990s improved *some* conditions for *some* women, but care, which previously had been universal, had become unequal in terms of quality and accessibility. Neither women nor practitioners could improve the conditions in which maternity care was provided or received. In order to address these challenges, the State initiated a new set of reforms at the turn of the century, denoted by social scholars as "the Statist turn" in Russian welfare policy. On the one hand, this turn denoted the new rhetoric of the State and its demographic concerns (see later). On the other, the actual ways in which these policies were implemented stimulated both neoliberalization and the reproduction of the top-down paternalistic approach. This mix of processes that shaped the current institutional pattern of Russian healthcare constitutes what we call *hybridization*. The following section focuses on the particular reforms that considerably influenced this process.

Reforms from the mid-2000s: the demographic ideological concern

The post-Soviet transformations in maternity care are to a large extent a top-down process induced by the new State's pronatalist agenda. In 2006, President Putin proclaimed the demographic objective of population growth as a priority task of the State, and offered a number of support measures for mothers and babies (President of Russia, 2006). Thereby, the State ranked demography, fertility and maternity care higher than they used to be in Russian policies and politics. The quality of maternity care was meant to be connected to the State's primary interest in population growth. The ongoing pronatalist rhetoric was followed up by certain practical steps. Since 2006, ideological and institutional reforms under this pronatalist agenda have consisted of ongoing social programs and have led to the State's attempts to modernize and rearrange maternity care in order to improve its quality and accessibility (Ministry of Health, 2012).

As Ginsburg and Rapp (1995) clearly showed, childbirth is always a political issue because it is all about reproducing and expanding or limiting the various populations within a given nation and, thus, is inevitably a part of the symbolic, gendered, racialized and moral order involved in the State's political agenda (see also Rivkin-Fish, 2006, 2010; Chernova, 2008; Zdravomyslova & Temkina, 2011, pp. 28–29; about Soviet society, see Nakachi, 2021; Leykin & Rivkin-Fish, 2022). Nation-states have long made efforts to expand the growth of their desired populations and to limit or stop the growth of "undesirable" populations (Ginsburg & Rapp, 1995). The Russian government's interest in childbirth reflects its desire for a population increase as an issue of State security.

The policy announced a goal to overcome the considerable decrease in both population growth and the childbirth rates of the 1990s (Vishnevsky, 2012, pp. 8–10). Special attention was given to maternal and perinatal mortality rates. Demands and standards came from the State bodies and were explicitly and implicitly formulated in the 2000s and put into practice via reforms in maternity care and, more broadly, by the State's demographic policies (Rivkin-Fish, 2010, p. 702; Cook, 2011, p. 14). The State framed the conditions of maternity care as the main providers of both healthcare services and societal growth (Cook, 2011; Chernova, 2013b; Borozdina et al., 2019). The governmental "care" of women was and still is limited to the cohort that has small children or at least a reproductive potential – they get social support and become "patronized" by the State, which tried to "stimulate births" by implementing extensive reforms.

Since 2006, ideological and institutional initiatives under this pronatalist agenda have consisted of the ongoing social program of so-called "maternity capital," in the form of non-recurrent payments to mothers who give birth to a second or subsequent child (Borozdina et al., 2016), a "childbirth vouchers" program (discussed in detail later on) and alterations to maternity care policies (e.g., monthly allowances for low-income families equal to the subsistence minimum). Demographic concerns have led also to the State's attempts to modernize and rearrange maternity care in order to improve quality and accessibility (Ministry of Health, 2012).

On the one hand, these reforms coincided with the demand for more woman-centered care arising bottom-up (from women and their families). But on the other hand, these reforms were widely criticized for insufficiency. Therefore, paradoxically, the state's financial investments were greeted positively, but they didn't reach their goal of sufficiently increasing population growth (Chernova, 2013a, b; Biryukova & Sinyavskaya, 2021). Families noticed that the provided state resources were not enough to cover their financial needs and that their own resources could not cover the expenses of having more children (which are quite high). In other words, the financial investments of the State did not sufficiently change the reproductive strategies of families in ways that ensured greater population growth. Thus, its demographic concerns have led to the State's attempts to modernize and rearrange maternity care in order to improve its quality and accessibility (Ministry of Health, 2012).

Reforms from the mid-2000s: the marketization of health and maternity care

The most significant reforms were launched in the mid-2000s. Since 2006, the State's political course has changed from a liberal to a more Statist one (Cook, 2011) – in other words, the State declared its (paternalistic) responsibility for public health. In 2006, the federal government initiated a "Foreground National Project 'Health'," which included increased funding to reproductive health services and some borrowings from market principles. One of the instruments developed to increase competition among medical institutions that provide care for women and children was a program called "Childbirth vouchers" (*rodoviye sertifikaty*), which provided the possibility for women to choose – within the free mandatory medical insurance – the institution for outpatient obstetric care (monitoring of pregnancy), childbirth and monitoring of children during the first year after birth. This system also allowed childbearing women to choose which obstetrician (but not a midwife) to consult with during pregnancy within the chosen facility (Borozdina & Titaev, 2011). The birth facility that gets a voucher from a woman receives a certain amount of money from the social security fund. While the territorial principle is still enacted (as it is more comfortable for most women to go to the closest facility), medical institutions have become more interested in attracting patients in order to get additional payout via these vouchers.

With the introduction of the childbirth vouchers, which implemented the principle "the money follows the woman," hospitals could partially improve their conditions. The revenues from this program were forwarded to the improvement of the material and technical conditions and an increase in providers' salaries (Ministry of Health and Social Development, 2005). Special financial stimulations for hospitals and healthcare providers were introduced in accordance with neoliberal market principles – hospitals were forced to attract more patients by offering them better care. Childbearing women received choices that had not previously existed, and that did not involve payments or informal agreements, however on a limited spectrum.

This kind of marketization was paradoxically intended to make health providers more patient (women)-oriented, but *not* less State-oriented. Providers continue to be dependent on the rigid standards and contradictory requirements of the controlling bodies. The current maternity care system remains paternalistic but implements quasi-market components. Financial investments from the State and funds attracted from women have allowed significant improvements in infrastructure and supply. Zhenya, an obstetrician aged 52, describes some of the marketing changes in her state-funded hospital, which has improved physical conditions and arranged some additional services:

> *Before that [the renovation, which happened within the framework of the 'Health' Project] there were no single rooms [for childbirth]. There were big rooms, which were designed to include four women . . . there were no single rooms. Naturally, there were no luxury rooms* [now there are]. *Now in the postnatal ward there are rooms for five women at maximum, but mostly for two-three.*

Such changes affect not only material and institutional settings for childbirth but also the format of social interactions and women's expectations concerning the spectrum and the quality of maternity services. As a result, relationships between patients and providers became more consumeristic, women became more demanding in their consumer needs, and providers had to adapt themselves to market logic. We will analyze this situation in more detail in Chapters 4 and 5.

Reforms from the mid-2000s: centralization and inconsistencies in maternity care

In the 2000s, the Russian Ministry of Health implemented centralized politics of maternity care improvement, which incidentally led to reduction in care quality and accessibility in remote areas. All maternity hospitals and departments were divided into a three-level system according to the amount and complexity of services, equipment, beds and specialists available at each facility. Level 1 denotes the smallest childbirth clinics, which can assist with only normal physiologic births. Level 2 hospitals have Intensive Care Units (ICUs) and Neonatal Intensive Care Units (NICUs) and can provide help in situations of complicated pregnancies and births, such as performing cesarean birth.[2] Level 3 denotes hospitals that can provide the most advanced care, including highly technological help for mothers and newborns – such as technologies for feeding those born prematurely, performing operations on mothers and newborns, treating infants with congenital diseases and malformations (Ministry of Health and Social Development, 2009).

Childbearing women can be transferred from Levels 1 and 2 to Level 3 if risks of birth complications are estimated during their pregnancies. This principle of "routing" (*marshrutizatsia*) was designed to increase both the quality and accessibility of maternity care; and, further, this system has been constantly developing. The system defines the route of a patient from one level of care to another: in cases of need, childbearing women should be forwarded to the higher-level unit that is best equipped to deal with them or their baby's particular complication(s). This means that if a woman lives close to a Level 1 unit and plans to deliver there, but has some complications during pregnancy or birth, then she will be transferred to a second or third level unit. Federal facilities of Level 3b (Federal Perinatal Centers) are available for free only to those with certain clinical conditions (from any region of Russia); others have to pay for their services (if they want to give non-complicated birth there). In Chapter 6, we will illustrate the difficulties caused by this routing system to the practices of remote maternity care facilities.

Women can choose in which facility of Level 1 or 2 they want to give birth, and sometimes they can also choose which Level 3 facility they will be transferred to. In emergent situations, women will be transferred to the hospital that is on duty that day, specializes in such cases, or is the closest one. The Federal Perinatal Centers (Level 3b) usually accept women who got their referrals ("quota") to hospitalize there in advance, after a medical commission qualifies her case as deserving the most advanced care. A "treatment quota" is the amount of money allocated from the State budget to the medical facilities to cover high-technological health services provided to its citizens. This sum is limited to a year, so the provision of medical care under a quota can be carried out only for a certain number of patients, which leads to the formation of queues for receiving such services.

Here we provide an example of how this routing model shaped the personal trajectory of a pregnant woman who lives in a remote region approximately 12 hours by air from a Level 3 hospital:

> *During the first screening on 31st week antenatally in our remote region, we [the fetus] were diagnosed with inborn heart disease. . . . It was a shock, it was scary, I was vomiting all the time . . . Thus, we didn't ourselves decide where to give birth – we went to the place where we got the quota, where we were referred to by our region. . . . If the disease had been diagnosed later, we would have been referred to [another big city, 6 hours of flight], because our region is working with them. . . . Then I was struggling for referral, so to say. I entered a queue, there were some big troubles with these documents. All in all, we had been waiting for an answer from [hospital] for a very long time, whether they will take me for delivery or not. . . . Some month and a half. Because they had to make a Concilium [at our region]. And on the 35th week we flew to [the city].*
>
> (interview with Alisa, mother, age 32)

Alisa's story demonstrates that the opportunity to choose the place of birth can be a struggle for mothers-to-be, as they face multiple organizational and logistical challenges in following the route of hospitalization. The reasons that made Alisa worry were: 1) the limited number of quotas and the non-transparent requirements for getting them; 2) Level 3 maternity units are mostly located in big cities, which are far away from her town; 3) there is not much time left before the due date. If she or her family has expectations or wishes that differ from the institutionalized track of routing, they must make additional efforts to organize an alternative path of monitoring and hospitalization. The success of such a plan depends not only on the routing scheme but also on the personal investments of time, management and money, in order to reach the hospital a woman or family has chosen. Problems of this kind are still quite common in the routing system, as maternity care within and across regions still remains highly inconsistent in terms of quality and even material conditions.

At the beginning of the 2010s, further reforms were implemented as a new program of "Modernization" was initiated at the Federal level. This program included measures aimed at the technological development of medical care in Russia through additional state subsidies given to public institutions to purchase new equipment and to raise state employees' salaries. Within the framework of this program, more Level 3 facilities were opened or rearranged in some regions (Government, 2013). These centers are supposed to head the system of maternity care within each region of the country. However, not all the regions could financially afford to construct such facilities; thus, several regions simply designated the largest maternity hospitals in those regions as Level 3, even when they didn't actually fully fit the criteria.

The higher the assigned level, the more financial support and equipment a maternity facility receives. This system of care provision has led to relatively unfavorable conditions for lower-level maternity care facilities (we return to this subject in Chapter 6). They do not have sufficient resources to attract more patients and have to route some risky cases to higher-level facilities, thereby losing the money that every such patient could bring. This form of the organization of maternity care created problems for the residents of remote areas, where accessibility to care has worsened, as Level 3 facilities are located exclusively in large cities. Unevenness of accessibility and quality of maternity care have been aggravated by another process – the closure of "FAPs" (*feldshersko-akusherskiye punkty*) – small medical facilities providing only paramedical services (and basic midwifery), located in villages and rural areas. This process of closure of some health and maternity care facilities was framed as a policy of "optimization" – that is, the reallocation of material and social resources. This process was not formalized as an independent State policy; however, in fact, it proceeded in parallel with the State programs, which have been taking the "Statist turn" since 2006. The shrinkage of maternity care in peripheral areas is not specific to Russia; there is evidence of the same process in other countries (Baillot & Evain, 2013; McCourt et al., 2016). However, this case in Russia signifies the ideological inconsistency between the State's rhetoric and actual policy implementation, as well as another round of the hybridization of regulatory logics.

The quality and accessibility of health and maternity care was planned to be improved by increasing the salaries of state-paid medical providers within the framework of "Modernization." This program was intended to rely on finances from regional budgets, which are quite limited. As a result, the numbers of medical practitioners were reduced in the smallest facilities located in remote areas (Starodubov & Sukhanova, 2013; Barkovskaya et al., 2013). Another consequence was that instead of increasing their salaries, many facilities increased working hours for maternity care providers and staff; thus, the prescribed indicators of income were reached by overloading the personnel. Regulations were aimed exclusively at "medical practitioners." Therefore, some nursing assistants and nurses were officially demoted into *sanitarki* (cleaners), who are counted as non-medical practitioners. They lost their status (which was symbolically important) and often were paid less than they would have been had their previous positions been preserved. All these measures were aimed at producing a picture showing that the average salaries of "medical practitioners" at hospitals (including maternity ones) seemingly grow, but this picture descended into dissatisfaction and worsening of working conditions in facilities that didn't receive enough finances to execute the Presidential decrees.

One further innovation was the modernization of the Mandatory Health Insurance (Federal Law, 2010). The financing of healthcare services has changed to the "one-channel" model, presupposing that all healthcare facilities receive money only through MHI, without any supplementary subsidies from regional authorities, as used to be the case (Shishkin et al., 2015;

Shuvalova et al., 2015). In some cases, this has led to insufficient financing, as MHI tariffs to a large extent depend on the size of the previous year's financing and do not relate to actual needs. As a consequence, the real expenditures in different regions and in different institutions vary considerably (Shishkin et al., 2016, p. 51). This led to more cutbacks in financing and in the number of healthcare workers.

As a result of these multi-stage reforms, the Russian system of maternity care has proceeded down a path of change and come up to the current arrangement, which is shaped by both the legacy of the Soviet centralized system of coordination and the neoliberal principles of supply and demand. The following section will specifically address the interweavings of these regulatory logics and the contradictions on the organizational and interactional levels that they have caused.

Contradictory results of health and maternity care transformations

The results of State reforms and their consequences for healthcare provision are contradictory. Maternity care was sufficiently improved in terms of technology, comfort, the number of services available and the qualifications of care providers – especially in perinatal centers and other large maternity hospitals. Women received the possibility to choose their birthing facility, and maternity wards became more open, as officially, partners were allowed to attend births (although this is still limited in practice), and providers became more patient-centered. However, the State still does not meet the demands and expectations of pregnant women or meets them only to a certain extent. According to sociological surveys, both healthcare providers and receivers in Russia negatively evaluated the results of these reforms. In particular, they complained that the latest reforms caused deteriorations in healthcare financing, increases in healthcare providers' workloads and cutbacks in facilities and personnel (Levada-center, 2016, pp. 23, 26).

Healthcare managers and experts have also evaluated the results of recent reforms pessimistically. Statistical analysis shows that "the introduced programs of financial support, although rather generous, cannot provide the increase in fertility rates inscribed in national programs and plans" (Biryukova & Sinyavskaya, 2021, p. 65). In sum, scholars who study this problem agree that, along with certain improvements, at a wider scale, these reforms have failed; as Rugol et al. (2018, p. 2) put it: "reforms aimed at improving healthcare (maternity care included), effectiveness, strengthening its infrastructure, improving conditions in medical organizations quality of medical care, and health of the population have failed to achieve the targets."

Regarding maternity care, this means that the liberal changes of the 1990s proceeded unsystematically and were accompanied by "shadow," or hidden, economic practices (Shishkin, 2003; Cook, 2014) such as the informal payments, which still have not left the scene. Later, in the early 2000s, the system was subject to the "Statist" turn in welfare policy, meaning an increase in the State's ruling paternalistic role in regulating and financing maternity care, and simultaneously an oxymoronic attempt to create market incentives under financial cutbacks and new principles of healthcare provision. As we have seen, the reforms limited access to medical services in remote areas and made the situations of some vulnerable groups of both maternity care receivers and providers in the rural facilities even more precarious.

For all health and maternity care providers, working conditions have changed, and rules (formal and informal) have become more complicated (see Chapter 5). The number of hospital beds and personnel was reduced (Ministry of Health, 2015), while the number of patients did not change accordingly. This "optimization" led to increases in workloads for the physicians, midwives and nurses who remained. Formally articulated policy goals of care improvement are often contradicted by actual outcomes. We agree with Meri Kulmala and her colleagues, who claim that "federal policies that appear at first glance to be neoliberal or statist might actually function through very different logics locally" (Kulmala et al., 2014, p. 540), and add that there is no linear path of change in the field of maternity care in Russia, but rather a hybridization of multiple institutional logics that result in contradictory policies, as explained in the next section.

As a result of the reforms, the current structure of maternity services has changed since the Soviet model, although it still exhibits its Statist and paternalist way of regulation (Shuvalova et al., 2015). Healthcare providers suffer a considerable bureaucratic burden of paperwork and statistical reporting (Romanov & Yarskaya-Smirnova, 2011; Levada-Center, 2016; Barskova et al., 2018), and the healthcare system in general and maternity care in particular are centrally regulated, not via professional associations with professional autonomy (such as the American College of Obstetricians and Gynecologists), but in a top-down manner, via the Ministry of Health and other State bodies. Thus, by the beginning of the 2020s, both the marketing and managerial principles of regulation have been implemented in maternity care, producing multiple institutional inconsistencies, which we address in the final section of this chapter.

Rule inconsistencies and practical discrepancies in Russian maternity care

Our next tasks are to explain why implemented State policies often do not work in the way they are designed to and why this causes problems for the performance of the System on both institutional and practical levels. Emerging institutional inconsistencies restrict the possibilities for improving the quality of maternity care. To explore this on a practical level, we will first describe the typical route of a childbearing woman in the landscape of maternity care in order to show its discontinuities. Next, we will analyze the multiple regulatory rules that shape the work of medical institutions, in order to highlight their inconsistencies.

The medicalized route of a pregnant woman in Russia: discontinuity of care

In this section, we describe the trajectory of a pregnant woman within maternity care in order to illustrate the heterogeneity of this institutionalized field, both at societal and organizational levels. The organization of maternity care in Russia is characterized by several key features. Among these are technologization and medicalization, with the risk-oriented model at the core. As we have seen, the Russian maternity care system is highly centralized, with uneven distribution of accessibility and quality across and within different facilities and regions, especially in the center-periphery/urban-rural dimension (Panova, 2019, p. 178). Different rules in different units with different resources often contradict each other, and childbearing women have to deal with these contradictions and their resultant discontinuities of care.

We note again that, by law, maternity care for pregnant women is free-of-charge, covered by the mandatory health insurance (MHI). The route of a pregnant woman today to a large extent resembles the route during the Soviet period. The commercial sector of delivery care is developing rapidly, but mostly women either use free-of-charge services or combine services provided by MHI with out-of-pocket payments. Despite the track chosen, all women have to register their pregnancies (*vstat' na uchet*) at a facility licensed for this (all State-funded and some private ones). There are certain stimulations for women to register early – they receive a small payout if they register before 12 weeks, and registration before 20 weeks of gestation in some regions provides an additional cash benefit after birth. To register, a woman usually goes to a "women's consultation" (prenatal and gynecological clinic), visits an obstetrician and a midwife and undergoes numerous tests and check-ups. After her first visit, she gets a document – an "exchangeable card" (*obmennaya karta*) – which she has to bring with her to all visits and which contains all the medical information about the course of her pregnancy; she must provide this card when she goes to a maternity hospital to give birth or gets other medical help during pregnancy.

Childbearing in Russia remains primarily oriented toward monitoring risk factors by obstetricians and other physicians in medical settings. During the course of her pregnancy, every woman has to consult with many doctors and undergo many tests: regular blood and urine tests, swabs for infections and a minimum of three ultrasounds. She can also get consultations with the staff psychologist and attend courses for parents-to-be, if they are available in the women's consultation she is assigned to. The Ministry of Health (2012) prescribes, as a minimum for a physiologic pregnancy, not less than seven appointments with an obstetrician-gynecologist, two with a general practitioner, two dental check-ups, one ophthalmological and one otorhinolaryngological appointment. In addition, pregnant women must have ultrasound diagnostics and HIV, syphilis, and hepatitis tests every trimester. Women with pregnancy complications receive extra consultations with physicians, who can recommend technologically advanced prenatal care without additional payments. By law, a neonatologist must attend all deliveries, including those in the Level 1 facilities (Ministry of Health, 2012). In case of complication, including cases of cesarean births, an anesthesiologist, surgical nurse and other specialists are to attend the delivery as well (ibid.). After her hospital delivery, a woman usually stays there at least for three days (if her birth was normal), and then she will be visited at home by a "patronage nurse" and a pediatrician, who will monitor her newborn every few days during the first month, and then monthly in a clinic during the first year.

All the services described earlier are guaranteed and covered by mandatory health insurance, while the paid services offer almost the same route, with some options of more comfort and better quality of care. For instance, the presence of a partner is allowed at "free" births, but only if there are no other women in that birth room. Payment for a personal room guarantees privacy and the possibility for the partner to participate. Commercial services provide possibilities for longer obstetrical visits, more comfort and the option of choosing the care provider. The range of choice is much wider in large cities, while in rural and remote areas, even access to free-of-charge facilities can be limited (due to the previously mentioned facility closures). In these cases, women are recommended to plan their visits and go to the hospital well in advance of the start of labor.

Thus, numerous providers and facilities are responsible for the health of a mother and a newborn. In practice, this situation leads to the lack of continuity of care, and women often face discoordination in the approaches of physicians in women's consultations, private clinics, specialized centers, and public maternity hospitals. These providers have different backgrounds and resources, while local protocols vary across the hospitals and different units within them. Women have to adapt themselves to different local conditions and medical tactics when they move from one unit to another, or from one care provider to another, or between departments within the same facility. The work in each of these various units is managed manually and requires a lot of negotiations between providers (see Chapter 5); therefore, different facilities are generally poorly coordinated with each other, and sometimes have conflicting views on the same problems or aspects of gestation or birth. Within the same maternity facility, practitioners from different departments and units, despite formally having the same specialization and general instructions, quite often practice different approaches to maternity care. If a woman tells one obstetrician that another obstetrician (or general practitioner) gave her other prescriptions or recommendations, she will often hear:

"*I am not interested in what the other doctor says to you.*" Our interlocutors told endless stories of such discoordination, when they not only get different recommendations from different physicians but also poorly understand how to receive service if they need to visit another physician or take additional tests. For instance, they might still need to come personally in the morning to clinic and queue to make an appointment, while number of available appointments is very limited. Although the System is becoming more digitalized, in some places things remain just as the way they used to be in the Soviet facilities. Therefore, many women prefer to pay for visits or check-ups in private clinics in order to avoid complicated navigation across different public institutions. Paternalistic concerns are persistent, not only on the level of State policy and regulation but also at the micro-level of practitioner-patient communication. Thus, the starting point of the present Russian system of maternity care – the Soviet System – has developed into an institution that remains to a high degree complicated, non-transparent/opaque and discoordinated, despite the multi-stage rearrangement that it went through.

The inconsistency of hospital rules

We conceptualize the institutional inconsistency of rules for maternity care as the contradictions of different *institutional regulatory logics*, following the concept introduced by the sociologist of professions Eliot Freidson (2001). According to Freidson, *professionalism* is only one of three regulatory logics in organizational fields; the other two are *marketing* and *bureaucracy*. These latter two challenge the idea of autonomous professional practice and restrict professional agency, which Freidson finds unfavorable, as only professionals fully know how to accomplish clinical tasks in an appropriate way. As other researchers have developed this idea:

> organizational fields are characterized by institutional complexity, comprising multiple logics, as opposed to being dominated by a single logic. In addition, these multiple logics may be competitive, but their relationship may also be co-operative, orthogonal, or blurred.
>
> (Currie & Spyridonidis, 2016, p. 78)

In the Russian context, these three logics coexist: medical professionals act simultaneously as state employees (managerial/bureaucratic logic), as service providers for patients-as-consumers (market logic) and/or as relatively autonomous decision-makers (professional logic). Mostly, they have to combine different rules in order to make their conditions workable. This leads to systematic contradictions, as the State often generates rules that, in practice, do not take into account the marketing principles of health and maternity care provision nor the professional (clinical) ones. Maternity care practitioners are often confused about which demands are primary for them. In the context of post-Soviet transformation, such hybridization is additionally framed by State systematic intervention (a post-Soviet paternalism), which is partially compensated for by informal horizontal networks in which participants informally negotiate rules and make personal decisions about them ad hoc (as fully discussed in Chapter 5).

The Hospital we studied is a Level 3 facility; these are the most complicated in terms of institutional structure, have the widest set of services and accumulate the most complicated childbirth cases. Therefore, the probability of bad clinical outcomes here is much higher than in lower-level maternity facilities. A Level 3 Hospital also symbolically and institutionally represents the cutting edge of medicalized and technologized maternity care in Russia, and hence is a subject of even more increased State interest and control (see Litvina et al., 2020). Being the most technologically developed and among the largest maternity facilities in the country, and providing multiple medical services, the Hospital has a complex organizational structure, which requires systematic coordination within the facility and with other organizations from different regions of the country. The Hospital includes more than a dozen wards and departments, and hundreds of practitioners and technical staff. At the same time, it is a part of a much bigger clinical complex. In practice, this setup considerably increases the need for coordination among different providers and the work of obstetricians, other physicians and managers, using up their resources of time and attention. Practitioners mostly cooperate with each other in a personal, informal way in order to solve current problems and needs. Paradoxically, the more complex the organization, the more rules participants have to obey and also the more informal work has to be done in order to manage inconsistencies. Systematic problems in coordination are inevitable, as rigid regulatory rules are unable to take into account every detail, every case and every clinical situation.

However, health and maternity care providers have little opportunity to affect top-down decision-making in the spheres of regulation, financing and the material provision of services at both societal and institutional levels. Even administrators of the Hospital complained that they could not pay enough to those who work long hours and are effective in their work. Some normative restrictions lead to confusing results, when, for example, purchased equipment cannot be used either due to poor quality, or absence of money to repair it, or there is no one skilled enough to work with it. Yet National State Programs (such as "Health" since 2006 or "Modernization" since 2011) encourage hospitals to make those kinds of purchases, as they symbolize high-tech progress and modernization.

The professional autonomy of obstetricians and other physicians has long been restricted by State paternalistic rulings and is now systematically challenged by marketization (the consumerization of patients and the commercialization of care) and managerial control. This chaotic and confusing situation has resulted in numerous multi-directive requirements and the expectations of different agents following differing institutional logics. This is how the head of one of the departments of the Hospital reflects on the inconsistent requirements, shaping the work of the unit (we will return to this story in Chapter 5, as it is very important):

> *We are unprotected from anyone [complaining patients and controlling State bodies]. Our [Hospital's] lawyer – I want to cry over him. If a mom wants to take the baby [get out of the Hospital before the therapy is over], should I give it? I don't know! This [absence of knowledge about the law] is such a colossal failure. We are not being taught what we should do. If a mom wants to change the physician, what should I do? I don't know. The local lawyer is incompetent. I hear him consulting with Google when I call him [with my practical questions]. . . . No one is going to defend us in court. Basic legal issues – we are to open the book of Civil Code ourselves. . . . Can a mom be responsible for a child if she is fifteen? I don't know, neither does the lawyer.*
>
> (field notes, interview with Valentina, head of department)

This field note illustrates that even maternity care providers (such as a department head) in a managerial position are not always aware of the legal regulations and other formal rules regulating maternity care. Valentina does not know how to behave when a mother wants to leave the hospital with a still-sick child or to change her physician, or the mother herself is a teenager. There is no office in the Hospital able to answer Valentina's numerous questions, nor are there transparent written rules. Her emotional narrative demonstrates that maternity care providers routinely find themselves between "the rock and the anvil" – between the patients' demands and the State's rigid regulations. Even the Hospital's lawyers are not competent in all the regulatory nuances that affect caregiving in this maternity hospital and others.

In our field site, we observed numerous contradictions between different rules, which confuse care providers and force them to adapt. We illustrate such contradictions and adaptive strategies through an obstetrician's narrative. Bureaucratic logic (of state-designed and controlled standards) affects the opportunity to act on the professional knowledge about a given clinical condition. Obstetrician Zhenya emphasizes the priority of the formal bureaucratic rules, which serve as the basis for the evaluation of her work and supposedly for the negative sanctioning of her personally or her department. Thus, she is forced to write information in a patient's medical record that differs from her real prescriptions in order to meet the formal standards, but in practice to follow her professional ideals of providing "good care":

> *So, the standards of care are introduced. If before that you could decide on your own what is best for a woman and her baby, now there are these standards. If you do the other way, you will be fired and punished. And if you do it the way you think is correct, you will either battle and defend it all . . . but then they won't let you work for a long time or you have to do it the way you think is right, but you have to write it down [into documents] the way it is supposed to be. That's why the record should be written "for the prosecutor".*

This quote reveals one of the ways in which the managerial logic of regulation (the necessity to follow the rigid standards imposed on medical practice that do not meet patients' needs) challenges the professional logic of autonomous decision-making, accomplished in accordance with the professional ideals of "good care." Such a conflict forces maternity care providers in some cases to falsify medical documents in order to meet the managerial standards and provide legal protection. Thus, Zhenya emphasizes that some medical documents are written not for a patient nor for a doctor, but for a law-enforcement body ("for the prosecutor").

The professional autonomy of obstetricians in decision-making about concrete cases is restricted by clinical recommendations and bureaucratic rules that require correct fill-in of all the documents. At the same time, such acts can be outdated or unspecific, and there are a lot of complaints about non-relevant protocols or clinical recommendations, which, according to our interlocutors, are often either translated from other languages without any adaptation or are written by a professor's assistant or student, as professors have no time. Anyway, as soon as this protocol becomes obligatory to follow, violating it can result in sanctions. Therefore, a regular practice of writing in the record about the treatment that *had to be done* instead of the one that *was actually done* (or writing down some indicators that are needed to satisfy the criteria for treatment prescription) is quite common, and patients sometimes are aware of that. Yet some physicians refuse to informally suggest more effective treatment (which is not listed in clinical recommendations and other regulatory documents) to patients, because there is always a risk of legal and financial prosecutions if such cases become evident.

Opaque or outdated rules lead to uncertainties that influence all participants, from maternity care providers to care receivers. The orientation toward fulfilling reporting requirements in medical practice leads to considerable bureaucratization: "The productive time of health practitioners' work is being reduced due to the growing and excessive paperwork, preparation of documentation and reports" (Shishkin et al., 2017, p. 15). Our interlocutors were constantly narrating about numerous "journals" (different sets of documentation reflecting the work of a medical institution, including various obligatory collected statistics):

> *[There should be 30 journals!] Not only mine, but in total [at the department]. I have a summary table, organizer and a calendar [to organize all the necessary data and information]! This is enough for me.*
>
> (field notes, interview with Valentina, head of department)

In the aforementioned citation, Valentina points at the mismatch in the number of journals her department *has to* fill in regularly (30) and the number of notebooks she *really needs* to organize her work (3). In other words, maternity care providers evaluate the amount of paperwork they are supposed to fill out as redundant. This situation is an indicator of the bureaucratic logic of regulation that dominates the Russian field of maternity care.

Women do not always recognize that their trajectory is often coordinated by very complicated personal efforts made by their care providers. Childbearing women emotionally react to all the organizational inconsistencies they notice, especially those associated with bureaucracy (when the provider had to follow the formal rules or was punished for not doing so):

> *We went to the hospital. But there was such a "wonderful" (sarcastically) man, . . . who refused to receive me. . . . Because I didn't have that reference . . . In short, I had to bring with me a reference saying that where I live [my home city, which is a 12-hour flight from the Hospital], there are no people diseased with tuberculosis registered there. . . . The point is that when they from the Hospital sent to our regional Ministry of Health a list of documents required for my hospitalization, the need for this reference was not mentioned. And I came without it. And he refused to receive me unless I bring this reference. It was a terrible experience, it was scary. Frankly speaking, there were lots of hysterics, lots of crying. . . . And via acquaintances, we found someone who would bring this reference to [the city].*
>
> (interview with Alisa, mother, age 32)

This quote illustrates that the excessiveness of documentation and paperwork shapes not only provider's work, but also patients' experiences. Although maternity care providers in some cases make efforts to compensate for the overbureaucratization of State-funded maternity care, it is still an extremely sensitive issue for the women receiving care. The ability to compensate for discontinuity of care and for the inconsistency of the formal rules – the System as we show in Chapter 6 – is vital for both maternity care receivers and providers. Informal practices, including those dealing with the formal requirements in manual personalized style, comprise important strategies in the negotiation of good care (for more on this, see Chapter 5).

Conclusion: inconsistency and discontinuity in Russian maternity care

The paternalistic Soviet system of maternity care was developed as a response to the demands of that time for free, public and accessible health and maternity care. It showed itself to be economically justifiable in terms of State interests, but was dissatisfying for both care providers and patients, including childbearing women, due to its opacity/non-transparency, low care quality, depersonalized relationships, State- rather than patient-orientation and the absence of choice and comfort. The first post-Soviet changes were fragmented and non-systematic, but were intended to overcome the disadvantages of the then-current system. And together with the problematization of the demographic situation – the low birthrates – at a higher governmental level, the reforms began full scale. The reforms of the 2000s took the pre-existing Soviet system as a basis; therefore, health and maternity care remained universal and free of charge, highly medicalized and centralized. At the same time, the State started to adopt new neoliberal market policies, which offered more rights and opportunities for women, and stimulated competition among hospitals and sometimes among care providers.

As we have shown in this chapter, those changes have had controversial effects. On the one hand, some hospitals could sufficiently increase the quality of their care and patients could get more choice and influence. On the other hand, these reforms negatively impacted vulnerable groups of patients living in remote areas and the personnel of small medical units, which couldn't meet the new standards due to their lack of financial viability and self-sufficiency.

Nowadays, Russian maternity care is characterized, first, by discontinuity of care, which childbearing women must deal with; and second, by the inconsistencies of rules in the hybrid combinations of professional, market and managerial logics and State paternalism, which all participants must deal with in medical institutions. Both care providers and care receivers elaborate strategies to deal with these challenges in order to improve maternity care. In the following chapter, we describe how childbearing women evaluate these changes and what they are currently demanding and receiving from Russia's troubled and overly complex maternity care system.

Notes

1 In Russia, neonatologists are professionals who specialize in working with babies during the neonatal period (up to 28 days). In addition, in maternity hospitals, they attend all births (including non-complicated ones) and monitor all newborn while they are getting in-patient services. There is also a sub-specialization called "resuscitator-neonatologist" – these are the specialists who work in NICUs

(Neonatal Intensive Care Unit). Pediatricians have a different specialization – they work with babies and children up to 18 years old and are not supposed to monitor newborns in maternity units.

2 The rate of cesarean birth in 2018 is 30% in Russian Federation (Ministry of Health of the Russian Federation, 2019).

References

Adonyeva, S., & Olson, L. J. (2011). Interpreting the past, postulating the future: Memorate as plot and script among Rural Russian women. *Journal of Folklore Research: An International Journal of Folklore and Ethnomusicology*, 48(2), 133–166.

Baillot, A., & Evain, F. (2013). Les maternités: un temps d'accès stable malgré les fermetures. *Journal de gestion et d'économie médicales*, 31(6), 333–347.

Barkovskaya, A. U., Huako, G. A., & Kamkin, E. G. (2013). Medicinskaya pomoshch' zhenshchinam v malyh gorodah Rossii [Medical care for women in small towns of Russia]. *Sociologiya goroda [City Sociology*], 1, 3–11 (In Russian).

Barskova, G. N., Lokhtina, L. K., Knyazev, A. A., & Zaporozhchenko, V. G. (2018). Otsenki vrachami optimizatsionnnykh izmeneniy v professional'noy deyatel'nosti [Doctors' evaluation of optimization changes in professional activity]. *Sotsial'nye aspekty zdorov'ya naseleniya [Social Aspects of Public Health]*, 64(6). Available at: http://vestnik.mednet.ru/content/view/1026/30/lang,ru/ (Accessed 16.06.2019) (In Russian).

Beloussova, E. (2002). The 'natural childbirth' movement in Russia: Self-representation strategies. *Anthropology of East Europe Review*, 20(1), 11–18.

Biryukova, S. S., & Sinyavskaya, O. V. (2021). More money – More births? Estimating effects of 2007 family policy changes on probability of second and subsequent births in Russia. *Monitoring of Public Opinion: Economic and Social Changes Journal* (Public Opinion Monitoring), 2.

Bogdanova, E. (2021). *Complaints to the Authorities in Russia: A Trap Between Tradition and Legal Modernization* (1st ed.). London: Routledge.

Borozdina, E. A. (2014). Yazyk nauki i yazyk lyubvi: legitimatsiya nezavisimoy akusherskoy praktiki v Rossii [Language of love and language of science: Legitimation of independent midwifery practice in Russia. *Laboratorium. Zhurnal sotsial'nykh issledovaniy* [*Laboratorium. The Journal of Social Studies*], 1, 30–59 (In Russian).

Borozdina, E. A., Rotkirch, A., Temkina, A., & Zdravomyslova, E. (2016). Using maternity capital: Citizen distrust of Russian family policy. *European Journal of Women's Studies*, 23(1), 60–75.

Borozdina, E. A., & Titaev, K. D. (2011). Sistema rodovykh sertifikatov: pravoprimenitel'nyye bar'yery v realizatsii reformy [The system of birth certificates: law enforcement barriers in the implementation of the reform]. *Seriya «Analiticheskiye zapiski po problemam pravoprimeneniya»* [Analytical notes on the problems of law enforcement]. enforcement], St. Petersburg: Institut Problem Pravoprimeneniya, EUSP. Available at: www.enforce.spb.ru/images/analit_zapiski/pm_1101_born.pdf (Accessed 14.11.18) (In Russian).

Borozdina, E. A., Zdravomyslova, E., & Temkina, A. (2019). *Sotsialnaya zabota: professii i instituty [Social Care: Professions and Institutions]*. St Petersburg: European University Press (In Russian).

Brown, J. (1987). The deprofessionalization of Soviet physicians: A reconsideration. *International Journal of Health Services*, 17(1), 65–76.

Chalmers, B. (1997). Changing childbirth in Eastern Europe: Which systems of authoritative knowledge should prevail? In R. Davis-Floyd & C. Sargent (Eds.), *Childbirth and Authoritative Knowledge: Cross-Cultural Perspectives* (pp. 263–286). Berkeley: University of California Press.

Chalmers, B. (2022). Teaching humanistic and holistic obstetrics: Triumphs and failures. In R. Davis-Floyd & A. Premkumar (Eds.), *Obstetric Violence and Syndemic Disparities: Can Obstetrics Be Humanized and De-Colonized*? New York: Berghahn Books, In Press.

Chernova, Z. (2008). *Semeynaya politika v Yevrope i Rossii: gendernyy analiz [Family Policy in Europe and Russia: Gender Analysis]*. Saint-Petersburg: Norma (In Russian).

Chernova, Z. (2013a). *Sem'ya kak politicheskiy vopros: Gosudarstvenniy proekt I praktiki privatnosti [Family as a Political Question: Governmental Project and Practices of Privacy]*. St. Petersburg: Izdatel'stvo Evropeyskogo Universiteta v Sankt-Peterburge [European University Press] (In Russian).

Chernova, Z. (2013b). New pronatalism?: Family policy in post-soviet Russia. *REGION: Regional Studies of Russia, Eastern Europe, and Central Asia*, 1(1), 75–92.

Cook, L. J. (2011). Russia's Welfare Regime: The shift toward statism. In M. Jäppinen, M. Kulmala, & A. Saarinen (Eds.), *Gazing at Welfare, Gender and Agency in Post-socialist Countries* (pp. 14–37). Newcastle upon Tyne: Cambridge Scholars Publishing.

Cook, L. J. (2014). 'Spontaneous privatization' and its political consequences in Russia's postcommunist health sector. In M. Cammett & L. M. MacLean (Eds.), *The Politics of Non-state Social Welfare* (pp. 217–236). Ithaca, NY: Cornell University Press.

Cook, L. J. (2017). Constraints on universal healthcare in the Russian federation: Inequality, informality and the failures of mandatory health insurance reforms. In Y. Ilcheong (Ed.), *Towards Universal Health Care in Emerging Economies* (pp. 269–296). London: Palgrave Macmillan.

Currie, G., & Spyridonidis, D. (2016). Interpretation of multiple institutional logics on the ground: Actors' position, their agency and situational constraints in professionalized contexts. *Organization Studies*, 37(1), 77–97.

Davis-Floyd, R. (2018). The technocratic, humanistic, and holistic paradigms of birth and health care. In R. Davis-Floyd (Ed.), *Ways of Knowing about Birth: Mothers, Midwives, Medicine, and Birth Activism* (pp. 3–44). Long Grove, IL: Waveland Press.

Davis-Floyd, R., & Cheyney, M. (2022). *Birth as an American Rite of Passage* (3rd ed.). Abingdon, Oxon: Routledge.

Federal Law. (2010). *No. 326-FZ "On Compulsory Health Insurance in the Russian Federation"*. Available at: www.garant.ru/news/1069288/#ixzz5X0Bz9m1E (Accessed 14.11.18).

Field, M. G. (1957). *Doctor and Patient in Soviet Russia*. Cambridge, MA: Harvard University Press.

Freidson, E. (2001). *Professionalism. The Third Logic. On the Practice of Knowledge*. Chicago: The University of Chicago Press.

Gaal, P., & McKee, M. (2004). Informal payment for healthcare and the theory of 'Inxit'. *The International Journal of Health Planning and Management*, 19(2), 163–178.

Ginsburg, F., & Rapp, R. (1995). *Conceiving the New World Order: The Global Politics of Reproduction*. Berkeley: University of California Press.

Government of the Russian Federation. (2013). *The Order "On Approval of the Program for the Development of Perinatal Centers in the Russian Federation"*. No. 2302-p of 09.12.2013. Available at: https://base.garant.ru/70529232/ (Accessed 19.07.22).

Jäppinen, M., Kulmala, M., & Saarinen, A. (2011). Introduction: Intersections of welfare, gender, and agency. In M. Jäppinen, M. Kulmala, & A. Saarinen (Eds.), *Gazing at Welfare, Gender and Agency in Post-socialist Countries* (pp. 1–12). Newcastle upon Tyne: Cambridge Scholars Publishing.

Kulmala, M., Kainu, M., Nikula, J., & Kivinen, M. (2014). Paradoxes of agency: Democracy and welfare in Russia. *Demokratiiya*, 22(4), 523–552.

Larivaara, M. M. (2010). Pregnancy prevention, reproductive health risk and morality: A perspective from public-sector women's clinics in St. Petersburg, Russia. *Critical Public Health*, 20(3), 357–371.

Levada-center. (2016). Protivostoyanie logik: vrach, patsient i vlast' v usloviyakh reformirovaniya sistemy zdravookhraneniya [Confrontation of the logics: doctor, patient and authority in the conditions of reforming the healthcare system]. *Svodnyy analiticheskiy otchet Tsentra Yuriya Levady* [*Summary Analytical Report of the Yuri Levada Analytical Center*]. Available at: www.levada.ru/cp/wp-content/uploads/2016/05/299_1-15_Svodnyj-analiticheskij-otchet.pdf (Accessed 16.06.2019) (In Russian).

Leykin, I. (2011). Population prescriptions: (Sanitary) culture and biomedical authority in contemporary Russia. *Anthropology of East Europe Review*, 29(1), 60–82.

Leykin, I., & Rivkin-Fish, M. (2022). Politicized demography and biomedical authority in post-soviet Russia. *Medical Anthropology Theory*, in print.

Litvina, D., Novkunskaya, A., & Temkina, A. (2020). Multiple vulnerabilities in medical settings: Invisible suffering of doctors. *Societies*, *10*(5). https://doi.org/10.3390/soc10010005.

McCourt, C., Rayment, J., Rance, S., & Sandall, J. (2016). Place of birth and concepts of wellbeing. *Anthropology in Action*, 23(3), 17–29.

Ministry of Health and Social Development of the Russian Federation. (2005). *The Order in "Childbirth Certificate"*. N 701 of 28.11.2005. Available at: http://www.consultant.ru/document/cons_doc_LAW_56881/ (Accessed 19.07.22).

Ministry of Health and Social Development of the Russian Federation. (2009). *The Order "On Approval of the Procedure for the Provision of Obstetric and Gynecological Care"*. N 808n of 2.10.2009. Available at: https://minzdrav.gov.ru/documents/7595-prikaz-minzdravsotsrazvitiya-rossii-808n-ot-2-oktyabrya-2009-g (Accessed 19.07.22).

Ministry of Health of the Russian Federation. (2012). *The Order "On Approval of the Procedure for Providing Medical Care in the Profile" Obstetrics and Gynecology (Except for the Use of Assisted Reproductive Technologies)*. N 572n of 1.11.2012. Available at: https://minzdrav.gov.ru/documents/9154-prikaz-ministerstva-zdravoohraneniya-rossiyskoy-federatsii-ot-1-noyabrya-2012-g-572n-obutverzhdenii-poryadka-okazaniya-meditsinskoy-pomoschi-po-profilyu-akusher-stvo-i-ginekologiya-za-isklyucheniem-ispolzovaniya-vspomogatelnyh-reproduk-tivnyh-tehnologiy (Accessed 19.07.22).

Ministry of Health of the Russian Federation. (2015). *Report on the State of Public Health and the Organization of Health on the Results of the Activities of the Executive Authorities of the Russian Federation in 2014*. Department of Monitoring, Analysis and Strategic Development of Health.

Ministry of Health of the Russian Federation. (2019). *The Key Indicators of Maternal and Child Health, the Activities of the Neonatal Care and Obstetric Services in the Russian Federation. Moscow.* Available at: https://minzdrav.gov.ru/ministry/61/22/stranitsa-979/statisticheskie-i-informatsionnye-materialy/statisticheskiy-sbornik-2018-god (Accessed 19.07.22).

Nakachi, M. (2021). *Replacing the Dead: The Politics of Reproduction in the Postwar Soviet Union*. Oxford and New York: Oxford University Press.

Novkunskaya, A. (2014). 'Bezotvetstvennyye' rody ili narusheniya norm rossiyskogo rodovspomozheniya v sluchaye domashnikh rodov ['Irresponsible' childbirth or contravention of Russian Midwifery's Norms in Homebirth cases]. *Zhurnal issledovaniy sotsial'noy politiki [Journal of Social Policy Studies*], 14(3), 353–366.

Ozhiganova, A. A. (2019). Official (biomedical) and alternative (home) obstetrics: Practices of formalized and informal interaction. *Economic Sociology*, 20(5), 28–52 (In Russian).

Panova, L. (2019). Access to healthcare: Russia in the European context. *The Journal of Social Policy Studies*, 17(2), 177–190 (In Russian).

Paton, C. R. (1989). Perestroika in the Soviet Union's health system. *BMJ: British Medical Journal*, 299(6690), 45–46.

President of Russia. (2006). *Annual Address to the Federal Assembly*. Available at: http://en.kremlin.ru/events/president/transcripts/23577/ (Accessed 13.09.2017).

Pushkareva, N. L., & Mitsyuk, N. A. (2017). The origins of medicalization: The basis of Russian social policy in the field of reproductive health (1760–1860). *The Journal of Social Policy Studies*, 15(4), 515–530. https://doi.org/10.17323/727-0634 2017-15-4-515-530.

Rivkin-Fish, M. (2005). *Women's Health in Post-Soviet Russia. The Politics of Intervention*. Bloomington: Indiana University Press.

Rivkin-Fish, M. (2006). From 'demographic crisis' to 'dying nation' – The politics of language and reproduction in Russia. In H. Goscilo & A. Lanoux (Eds.), *Gender and National Identity in Twentieth-Century Russian Culture* (pp. 151–173). DeKalb, IL: Northern Illinois University Press.

Rivkin-Fish, M. (2010). Pronatalism, gender politics, and the renewal of family support in Russia: Toward a feminist anthropology of 'maternity capital'. *Slavic Review*, 69(3), 701–724.

Romanov, P., & Yarskaya-Smirnova, E. (2011). Ideologii professionalizma i sotsial'noye gosudarstvo [Ideologies of professionalism and social state]. In P. Romanov & E. Yarskaya-Smirnova (Eds.), *Antropologiya professiĭ, ili postoronnim vkhod razreshen [The Anthropology of Professions, or Outsiders Allowed]* (pp. 64–82). Moscow: Variant LLC, TsSPGI (In Russia).

Rugol, L. V., Son, I. M., Starodubov, V. I., & Pogonin, A. V. (2018). Nekotorye itogi reformirovaniya zdravookhraneniya [Some results of the healthcare reform]. *Sotsial'nye aspekty zdorov'ya naseleniya [Social Aspects of Public Health]*, 64(6).

Available at: http://vestnik.mednet.ru/content/view/1023/30/lang,ru/ (Accessed 16.06.2019).

Saks, M. (2015). *Professions, State and the Market: Medicine in Britain, the United States and Russia*. Abingdon, New York: Routledge.

Sheiman, I., Shishkin, S., & Shevsky, V. (2018). The evolving Semashko model of primary healthcare: The case of the Russian Federation. *Risk Management and Healthcare Policy*, 11, 209–220.

Shishkin, S. V. (2003). Formal'nye i neformal'nye pravila oplaty medicinskoj pomoshhi [Formal and informal practices of healthcare services' payment]. *Mir Rossii: Sociologija, Jetnologija*, 12(3), 104–129.

Shishkin, S. V., Sazhina, S. V., & Selezneva, E. V. (2015). Izmeneniya v deyatel'nosti strakhovykh meditsinskikh organizatsiy v novoy sisteme OMS [Changes in the activities of health insurance organizations in the new OMS system]. *Obyazatel'noye meditsinskoye strakhovaniye v Rossiyskoy Federatsii [Obligatory Medical Insurance in the Russian Federation]*, 5, 32–37.

Shishkin, S. V., Sheyman, I. M., Abdin, A. A., Boyarskiy, S. G., & Sazhina, S. V. (2016). Rossiyskoye zdravookhraneniye v novykh ekonomicheskikh usloviyakh: vyzovy i perspektivy [Russian healthcare in new economic conditions: Challenges and prospects]. *Doklad NIU VSHE po problemam razvitiya sistemy zdravookhraneniya* [*HSE Report on the Problems of the Development of the Healthcare System*]. Moscow: HSE Publishing House.

Shishkin, S. V., Vlasov, V. V., Boyarskij, S. G., Zasimova, L. S., Kolosnicyna, M. G., Kuznecov, P. P., Ovcharova, L. N., Sazhina, S. V., Stepanov, I. M., Horkina, N. A., Shevskij, V. I., Shejman, I. M., & Yakobson, L. I. (2017). *Zdravoohranenie: sovremennoe sostoyanie i vozmozhnye scenarii razvitiya: dokl. k XVIII Apr. mezhdunar. nauch. konf. po problemam razvitiya ehkonomiki i obshchestva* [*Healthcare: Modern State and Possible Scenarios of Development: Paper for the XVIII International Conference on the Problems of Economic and Societal Development*]. Moscow, 11–14 apr. 2017 g. / Ruk.: S. V. Shishkin. Moscow: HSE Publishing.

Shuvalova, M. P., Yarotskaya, E. L., Pismenskaya, T. V., Dolgushina, N. V., Baibarina, E. N., & Sukhikh, G. T. (2015). Maternity care in Russia: Issues, achievements, and potential. *Journal of Obstetrics and Gynaecology Canada*, 37(10), 865–871.

Starodubov, V. I., & Sukhanova, L. P. (2013). Novyye kriterii rozhdeniya: mediko-demograficheskiye rezul'taty i organizatsionnyye problemy sluzhby rodovspomozheniya [New criteria for birth: Demographic and medical results and organizational problems of the obstetric aid service]. *Menedzher zdravookhraneniya*, 12, 21–29.

Stepurko, T., Pavlova, M., Gryga, I., & Groot, W. (2013). Informal payments for healthcare services–Corruption or gratitude? A study on public attitudes, perceptions and opinions in six Central and Eastern European countries. *Communist and Post-Communist Studies*, 46(4), 419–431.

Temkina, A. (2016). Oplachivaemaja zabota i bezopasnost': chto prodaetsja i pokupaetsja v rodil'nyh domah? [Paid care and safety: What is on purchase in maternity hospitals?]. *Sociologija vlasti [Sociology of the Power]*, 28(1), 76–106.

Twigg, J. L. (1998). Balancing the state and the market: Russia's adoption of obligatory medical insurance. *Europe-Asia Studies*, 50(4), 583–602.

Vishnevsky, A. G. (2012). Rossija: demograficheskie itogi dvuh desjatiletij [Russia: Demographic results of the two decades]. *Mir Rossii. Sociologija. Jetnologija [The World of Russia. Sociology. Ethnography*], 21(3), 3–40.

Younger, D. S. (2016). Health care in the Russian Federation. *Neurologic Clinics*, 34(4), 1085–1102.

Zdravomyslova, E., & Temkina, A. (2011). Doveritel'noe sotrudnichestvo vo vzaimodejstvii vracha i pacientki: vzgljad akushera-ginekologa [Trusting cooperation in doctor-patient interaction: Obstetrician-gynecologist's viewpoint]. In E. Zdravomyslova & A. Temkina (Eds.), *Zdorov'e i intimnaja zhizn'. Sociologicheskie podhody* [*Health and Intimate Life. Sociological Approaches*] (pp. 23–53). Saint-Petersburg: EUSP Publishing.

Chapter 4

Childbearing women in Russia

Consumer agency and the negotiation of "good care"

In this chapter, we present our empirical findings on childbearing women's practices, needs, expectations, and agency. We ask and answer the questions of what kinds of care women want and do not want to receive in maternity hospitals (the only legitimate setting in Russia for childbirth). We are interested in the changes in subjectivity of young Russian women, who in general have become more assertive, individualistic and consumer-oriented in comparison to previous generations, and in the concept of "good mothering" as transformed into "intensive mothering." We explore what strategies women implement in order to receive "good care," and how they are empowered (or not) during this process.

As we described in the preceding chapter, shifts in subjectivities and strategies take place under the influence of processes of consumerization and commercialization of health and maternity care. A key issue in worldwide debates on consumerism and marketization in healthcare is patients' choice as a part of a "rational actor" model focused on cultivating individual responsibility and agency (Temkina & Rivkin-Fish, 2020). However, as described in Chapter 3, in Russian health and maternity care, providers still sometimes have to place the interests of the State and the institution they work in over those of individual patients making choices. Hence, State control still dominates the field of maternity care, while market regulation is limited. In the Soviet and, to a large extent, the post-Soviet system, both care providers and receivers lack autonomy in decision-making, though in differing ways, and it is still expected that women in childbirth should submit themselves to obstetricians, who by law are held personally responsible for maternal health and childbirth outcomes and are controlled by numerous official State bodies.

Given that recently patients, as active consumers, have increased their demands concerning maternity care, in this chapter we ask to what extent those demands are being met by the provision of women-friendly services and women's empowerment. Our next question regards how women act if they do not receive attention to their needs and the emotional support they expect; we show that some of these actions involve posting complaints and

DOI: 10.4324/9781003139539-4

critical reviews on websites. Increasing consumer demands and complaints cause special challenges for maternity care providers, who must deal with these in the context of organizational uncertainties and must *manually manage* multiple institutional inconsistencies (as we explain in Chapters 3 and 5).

Demands from below: women's needs and strategies in maternity care

Here we explore how new women's demands and choices have emerged in the course of the reformation and commercialization of health care. We address what women are doing in order to cope with institutional uncertainties and to avoid the (post-)Soviet legacy of neglect, and how they work to establish trust with their care providers. We also question whether these new needs and new subjectivities have led to the reduction of paternalism in maternity care.

From the Soviet informalities to the post-Soviet market: women's choices

As described in the preceding chapter, in Soviet maternity care, childbearing women had to have their pregnancies monitored by an obstetrician and give birth in a specific State-funded medical institution without any alternative. Informal networks were the only ways through which they could positively affect their care (see Chapter 3). Pregnancy and childbirth in Soviet times, as well as in contemporary Russia, were and remain highly medicalized, with childbearing women perceived and treated as patients, and mostly not as consumers or clients. In the Soviet era, such social roles shaped the relationships between obstetricians as paternalistic State employees and the powerless and passively obedient childbearing women. *Khamstvo* (rudeness) – a type of emotional and verbal abuse (Temkina et al., 2021; Novkunskaya et al., 2020; Chapter 5) was a typical communicative practice that medical providers applied as an instrument for disciplining childbearing women during their pregnancies and births. Soviet women had little ability to reverse these positions and mostly had to obey clinicians and hope for a lucky outcome.

However, as previously noted, many women tried to avoid the traumatic experience of childbirth in Soviet hospitals by mobilizing their social networks. This informal system embraced *blat* – personal referral and informal agreements, and *bribes* – informal out-of-pocket payments. Women used to engage in these practices in order to find an obstetrician who could provide better, more personalized care and to decrease the probability of *khamstvo*. The centralized socialist maternity care system was partially balanced by this informal system (Rivkin-Fish, 2005; Stepurko et al., 2013; Cook, 2017). This system began to transform, along with the reforms that were aimed at the improvement of maternity care (described in Chapter 3) and at the legalization of unofficial payments via the childbirth vouchers (see Temkina & Rivkin-Fish, 2020).

The new market mechanisms and processes emerging in post-Soviet maternity care (ibid.; see also Temkina, 2019) were stimulated both by the State's financial limitations and women's demands. The Soviet model of universal public and free-of-charge maternity care services remains as a basis, but during the last three decades has been complemented with commercial facilities and paid services within public institutions (*platniye uslugi*). These paid services include the options to choose an obstetrician and – rarely – a neonatologist and midwife, get extra consultations (longer and with the physician of one's choice), partnered delivery, more comfortable rooms, etc. Jointly with a few private maternity hospitals, such paid services form a new, relatively small private sector of maternity care, which, however, is not actually separate from the public sector and is mostly based on it and regulated by the same orders. Over the last few years, we have also observed the emergence and growth of the marketing of commercial maternity care services provided by non-medical specialists, such as lactation consultants and doulas (for more details see also Chapters 5 and 6).

These neoliberal tendencies have resulted in the emergence of new consumer-like relationships between maternity care providers and recipients. Affluent women who pay for maternity care are more interested in receiving "good care" (Borozdina, 2016; Temkina, 2019; Temkina & Rivkin-Fish, 2020). As a result, there is much more "positive" emotional work done in maternity hospitals today, and politeness and *smiling* are promoted there (we will analyze these behaviors in Chapter 5). Affluent women officially pay the hospital in order to be cared for by chosen doctors and receive "good care" – or at least the kind of care that is closer to their expectations and desires. The higher class position of women who can afford such payments allows them also to benefit from personalized relationships of trust with concrete providers. Such relationships compensate to a certain extent for, and partially reduce, the discontinuity of care, institutional uncertainty and emotional suffering described in Chapter 3 (see also Borozdina, 2016; Temkina & Rivkin-Fish, 2020). Starting from the mid-2000s, all childbearing women in Russia (not only those who pay) received the possibility to choose a hospital according to their wish (Chapter 3). This option, stimulated by the neoliberal healthcare policies, created opportunities for new childbirth practices. The market segment in maternity care has become accompanied by broad shifts in modes of care, emotional styles (to be analyzed in the Chapter 5) and women's subjectivities.

The subjectivity of childbearing women in post-Soviet society

Rather than being obedient patients as in previous generations, childbearing women currently have become consumers, considering themselves free, assertive and aware of their needs; thus, a new type of post-Soviet subject has appeared within the shifting landscape of Russian maternity care. Childbearing women increasingly insist on being treated as clients, instead of as ignorant and vulnerable patients. They have become more vocal in expressing their needs and also more proactive agents in the constitution of a new institutional order and emotional style – a repertoire of performed emotional practices that characterize certain types of interaction in various institutional contexts in medicine (Temkina et al., 2021; Chapter 5). As a particular kind of service consumers, they actively seek the best care for themselves and their children.

The growth of women's demands is connected to the new commercialized and gendered practices of "intensive mothering" (Temkina, 2019; Temkina & Rivkin-Fish, 2020; Avdeeva, 2020). These new conceptions of motherhood presuppose intensive investment of resources in child-rearing. This "intensive mothering" involves consumer practices from the very beginning of pregnancy and even before conception (such as pre-conception diagnostics, regular visits to physicians, healthy lifestyle, courses and literature for future parents, home redesign, saving money for paid maternity care). Contemporary Russian women as responsible mothers have sufficient knowledge about pregnancy and delivery, hospitals and obstetricians, as well as certain ideas about "good care" and expectations of services they want to receive during pregnancy and delivery.

"Good mothering" in Russia (Hays, 1996; Utrata, 2015; Godovannaya & Temkina, 2017) implies a high degree of reflexivity, responsibility and financial investments. In line with the description of *intensive mothering* as "child-centered, expert-guided, emotionally absorbing, labor-intensive, and financially expensive" (Hays, 1996), young women believe in individual responsibility for the outcomes of their pregnancies and child-rearing. It is supposed that a "good mother" should be responsible for obtaining high quality of care during pregnancy, delivery and the postnatal period. Therefore, many mothers-to-be do not want to passively follow the prescribed impersonal institutional trajectory, nor place their hopes in the arms of fate, but prefer to take personal control over their perinatal experiences.

Women no longer accept that "doctor knows best"; they want to negotiate and receive "good care" according to their own expectations, which include support and attention to their needs and ideas about labor. Women have become sensitive to the quality of treatment, the style of communication and the emotional labor accomplished by care providers. They do not want to be treated within the Soviet-style *khamstvo* – impersonalized and rude – approach. Many women we interviewed said that they wanted to have control over the situation during pregnancy and labor:

> *[It is necessary] to really control every step, to be sure that you have done everything that you could do.*
>
> (interview with Agata, mother, age 31)

> *Everything should be controlled – hospital, doctor, it is necessary to choose beforehand.*
>
> (interview with Inna, mother, age 34)

According to our findings, childbearing women, as consumers and "good mothers," spend a lot of time and effort to generate "good care" during their pregnancy and childbirth, carefully making the "right choice" among the available options. Along with other issues, this process usually includes strategic seeking for "good care" and avoiding *khamstvo*.

Avoiding khamstvo *and looking for "good care"*

In their childbirth narratives, Russian women still quite often refer to their mothers' and grandmothers' experiences, framing them (and sometimes their own as well) as "horror stories" and stories about *khamstvo*. Such narratives consist of multiple details on poor conditions and the rudeness or neglect faced in maternity hospitals. A common refrain of these stories was articulated by one of our interlocutors: "*I read a lot about the horror of delivery in a corridor accompanied with the khamstvo of obstetricians*" (interview with Inna, mother, age 34). Women of the post-Soviet generation have tried to resist such Soviet-style maternity care and to act strategically to have a childbirth experience that is not, as one of our participants put it, "*like being on a conveyer, being alone and neglected in the corridor when all the wards are over capacity and there is no place*" (interview with Viktoria, mother, age 28).

The term *khamstvo* has come to convey the general atmosphere of women-unfriendly maternity services, which entails a general condition of dependency and helplessness. Our interlocutors identified *khamstvo* as a part of the Soviet legacy:

> *I had a boy (first child) in 1999, in an ordinary . . . Soviet maternity hospital, where there used to be ten people in the labor room. And the approach to a woman, you know . . . not as one appropriate for a woman experiencing suffering, torment, pain . . . Everything is managed as in [a conveyer line]. . . . Doctors shouted at me, and . . . they delivered my baby, but they did not provide any anesthesia! . . . I was giving birth for a very long time; it was so painful. So, in general, I was so tormented that I decided not to give birth again ever in my life.*
>
> (interview with Tamara, mother, age 44)

Tamara's statement illustrates the extreme levels of trauma that many women of that era experienced. Today, things that women want to avoid consist of: lack of attention or rudeness on the parts of physicians, nurses or midwives; the refusal to answer questions and explain the medical manipulations used; too many or too few medical interventions; incorrect clinical decisions made by obstetricians; changing of medical shifts in the midst of delivery without notification; discrepancies in the approaches of different providers; poor physical conditions (lack of toilets, showers, overcrowded wards, poor-quality food); the presence of other women in the delivery room; the inability to be accompanied by a partner; having the newborn taken away right after delivery; etc. In addition, our interlocutors did not want to follow the still-extant Soviet-style practice of calling an ambulance at the start of labor, which would take them in to "*an unknown hospital, in the hands of unknown experts*" (interview with Kira, mother, age 35). Childbearing women try to organize their childbirth and create their own systems of knowledge and preferences, which can help them to navigate in the Russian maternity care system, make the "right choice" and act in accordance with it.

Our interlocutors (both patients and some obstetricians) identified the Soviet-style approach to labor and birth as an "obstetric aggression" – or "obstetric violence," the same as it is called in many other countries (Sadler et al., 2016; Liese et al., 2021). In Russia, the term "obstetric aggression" (Radzinsky, 2011) indexes unreasonable and humiliating overmedicalized practices that can complicate birth and worsen a woman's physical and psychological state. Among these are obligatory shaving and enema before birth; the puncture of the amniotic sac (to "stimulate" birth); a prohibition on free movement during labor; refusal to provide epidural analgesia; unreasonable induction or augmentation of labor with artificial oxytocin; forcible separation or manual removal of the placenta (an excruciating procedure); Kristeller (manual pressure on the abdomen – a dangerous and now officially forbidden practice); and others. Many of these procedures are typical of medicalized births almost everywhere (see Davis-Floyd & Cheyney, 2019), yet in many high-resource countries, they are accompanied by humanistic touches, such as kindness and compassion on the part of caregivers (see Davis-Floyd, 2018). The same processes take place in Russia as well; in what Davis-Floyd (ibid.) calls "superficial humanism," some of the practices listed earlier are accompanied by caring behavior, whereas in Soviet-style birth, they were (and sometimes still are) accompanied by rudeness and often overt cruelty.

Childbearing women frequently repeated in interviews that they chose to pay for maternity care in order to ensure their emotional security and support. Women are afraid of being mistreated and want to "*avoid some boorish [khamsky] hardship . . . the things that happen in our [state-funded] maternity hospitals*" (interview with Kira, mother, age 35). Many interlocutors said that by paying for maternity services, they expected to receive more attention from their care providers: "*Everyone who participated in this process there, everyone did it with a smile, everyone was very kind, polite, pleasant*" (interview with Nina, mother, age 29). In these cases, emotional support is an extra paid work; Zoya, aged 28, described it as follows: *"[payment] gives a good attitude and respect, you buy respect for yourself during childbirth."* Another interlocutor, Svetlana, age 20, added, *"In principle, that's why I paid, in order to have . . . a respectful attitude . . . I read and was told [that labour] is not always a positive experience . . . emotionally . . . I decided that we should pay for my emotional safety as well."*

Women who make a deliberate choice to pay for childbirth care are especially interested in "warm care," meaning a kind and compassionate humanistic approach. This kind of care necessitates a change not only in communicative patterns but also in the physical environment, in the forms of separate rooms with individual toilet and shower, equipment for comfortable movement in labor (such as birthing balls) and pretty interiors. But the building of the needed infrastructure (spaces of care) is constrained by a number of factors and differs from hospital to hospital.

In searching for "good care," women compare their strategies with a market service: Alia, age 29, said, *"[This is] the same as staying in a hotel."* Women want to choose and receive "good care," but they understand it differently. For some, "comfortable conditions" are extremely important. They want to give birth in a separate room, together with their partner, and to have convenient conditions in the postpartum ward – all these options are mostly available only on a paid basis. And such women are ready to invest money in improving the conditions for their childbirth as they formulate their principle not to skimp on childbirth expenses. Other women say that the reputation of a doctor and/or emotional support matters most to them. They want to know their doctor or midwife in advance, and this is also available mostly on a paid basis. Such care includes emotional support for the laboring woman: *"When you give birth, you're scared. . . . You still do not know what is happening to you. And you want someone to hold your hand"* (interview with Marta, mother, age 31). The need to be "held by the hand" means the expectation of emotional work on the part of the care provider. Tais, age 30, says, *"But they must monitor . . . must be emotionally encouraging and watching so that everything is right."*

Consumers making "the right choice": seeking information

As we have just seen, today's Russian childbearing women are significantly less prone to suffer or just accept their fate than the women of the Soviet and early post-Soviet eras and are more likely to actively pursue their own initiatives. Young parents are becoming a particular kind of consumers who actively seek the best care for themselves and their children, engaging multiple financial and informational resources, including social media and networks. Social forums and media have become important sources of information for navigating through maternity care system and facilities. In particular, childbirth experiences with particular obstetricians and midwives and their styles of communication and emotional support are frequently discussed in detail online and in person. Mothers-to-be can make their choices among multiple options and so expect high-quality medical care that is "warm," professional and personalized. They seek respectful attention, support and comfortable conditions and also expect that professionals will not be cold and rude and will fulfill the emotional work of "holding by hand" women in delivery.

Antonina (age 40) took her search for information about childbirth and childbirth attendants so seriously that she even called it a "*kind of sociological survey*":

Q: *Please tell me how you are looking for such attendants?*
Antonina: *According to the recommendations. I have friends who have children. And I have relatives, doctors who are in this field. That is, I know more or less. I definitely use the internet. Of course. Be sure to read reviews, comments, and so on.*

Q: *What sites?*
Antonina: *I read different ones. I think the more information the better. Also a kind of sociological survey.*

Antonina describes her strategy for organizing paid childbirth as a series of well-designed and informed steps. She collected information from various sources, not trusting any of them without verification; based on this analysis, she selected two maternity hospitals suitable for her and formed her own opinion about their differences. In one case, more comfortable conditions were provided and a wide range of consumer services was offered; the quality of the labor rooms was similar to that of nice hotel rooms, and patients could choose their meals. In another maternity hospital, from Antonina's point of view, emergency care was more effectively organized, but it was impossible to book a specific postpartum room in advance. Well before her labor began, Antonina talked with the obstetricians who would assist with her labor, with an anesthesiologist, neonatologist and the head of the department, asked them questions about labor management, discussing their options, and listened to their arguments. She finally chose a suite room to labor and deliver in with her husband, signed a contract and officially paid for the provision of the services she opted for. During our interview, she emphasized that motherhood for her is a particularly significant experience, and when planning her birth, she did not set the goal of saving money (Temkina, 2018). Other women tell similar stories about their choices in the "market of maternity service":

> *I compared several places . . . with similar conditions, and with good reviews. We now always read reviews about everything. . . . And the*

> *money there, in fact, it turned out . . . more or less the same, because I was given a discount for being there.*
>
> (interview with Inna, mother, age 34)

When making a decision about paying for childbirth, women discuss this issue with their husband or partner; they calculate together what will be the burden on their family budget (for more details, see Temkina, 2017). Childbearing women as consumers try to resist to a certain extent the domination of medical knowledge and the expert power inherent in the technocratic model of childbirth (Davis-Floyd, 2001, 2003, 2018); they do not want to be ignorant and subject to an unknown fate any more:

> A *woman should know what childbirth is, know the stages of childbirth . . . We're always afraid of the unknown, [better] when you know what's going on with you, when you know what to do, when you know how to cope with pain, with your breath, when you know when to go to the shower, where to do hot water, where the lower back massage is [needed].*
>
> (interview with Regina, mother, age 35)

Women try to improve their knowledge in the fields related to the experience of pregnancy and childbirth in order to be prepared for the delivery and for infant care. Yet women who cannot pay privately for personalized care continue to perceive maternity hospitals as closed "black boxes" (semi-total institutions) with nontransparent rules, and obstetricians as anonymous representatives of the State, who make such women feel alone and neglected in a foreign and unfriendly environment. They cannot recall names and faces, do not understand the professional statuses of care providers who attend them, such as physicians of various specializations, nurses, midwives: "*What's their name? I don't know*" (online forum, for more details see Appendix 5).

Those who can pay for personalized care carefully collect relevant information. They investigate the organizational structure of the maternity care provided in the facility of their choice and the reputations of different obstetricians and midwives; monitor social networks and thematic groups; use special apps; read educational and medical sites; etc. For example, Alia, aged 29, found the forum "Littleone" to be especially helpful because there she could speak with experienced mothers who could give her helpful advice.

In forming their preferences, women collect information about the nuances of particular hospitals, especially when visiting a maternity hospital during an "Open Door Day" (some hospitals organize special events for all interested to visit and ask questions). Our interlocutors were aware that actual conditions in maternity hospitals and the approaches and attitudes of obstetricians may differ from those presented officially, and so they try to create a hierarchy of their preferences and learn more details about delivery in each facility.

During Open Door Day, future mothers and fathers ask a lot of questions: they want to understand how to get to this hospital; how the wards are equipped; how many hospital beds are there; where the toilets are located; how the regime of visits in paid and free wards organized; can a partner be present; whether the use of epidural analgesia is available; is it possible to have an elective cesarean birth (no, officially they can't); how many days postpartum will the new mother have to stay in the hospital; where a newborn is placed (kept with the mother or moved to a nursery); whether breastfeeding is taught; etc. They also find out when and how to sign a contract for paid services, whether it is possible to meet a midwife and obstetrician in advance, how much individual rooms cost (field note). In a separate study (Korotkikh & Popova, 2017), midwives listed the questions that childbearing women ask them when they meet: "Can I give birth naturally? How often is cardiotocography recorded during childbirth and is it possible to move at the same time? Is there a ball, a mat in the delivery room, is it possible to use a shower? Is it possible to refuse artificial labor induction or augmentation? Is it obligatory to give birth lying down? Will the newborn be put on my chest? How quickly will my newborn be attached to the breast? Will they remove the vernix from the newborn and drip an antiseptic into his eyes?" (ibid., pp. 27–28).

These and other questions are aimed at understanding the conditions in which childbirth and the postpartum period take place: what is the difference between paid and free services, how interventionist are obstetricians' actions during labor, whether a woman has the ability to refuse certain interventions, etc. Such questions demonstrate that women are quite informed and show not only their interest but also their awareness of the details of the medical management of the birthing process.

"Good care": personalization and construction of trust

However, "good care" could not be guaranteed even when numerous efforts were made, research was conducted and informed choice was made. Some childbearing women argued that only personalization of relationships guarantees trust as a prerequisite for "good care":

> *Most importantly, get to a doctor you know. That she was recommended, and preferably by some very close people. Relatives, for example.*
>
> (interview with Julia, mother, age 34)

> *These were already, of course, completely special conditions, because the doctor is really well known, and when he has been monitoring [pregnancy] for several months, yes, then such a rather trusting relationship* [is built].
>
> (interview with Oksana, mother, age 35)

Recall that in a typical case, in a (either free or paid) delivery in the State-funded hospital, a woman sees an obstetrician and a midwife for the first time when she enters the hospital to give birth, unless she had made an effort to get acquainted with them in advance.

The possibilities within the public maternity care system (covered by mandatory health insurance) are limited – it still functions like a conveyer belt aimed at processing a large number of patients. Therefore, standard regulations and overmedicalization determine care in such facilities. For instance, postnatal visits by relatives can be limited or even forbidden. There is a strict rule that children under 12 cannot enter hospitals to visit; and other visitors can also be denied access, especially in State-funded units, for "sanitary reasons." Moreover, new mothers can be denied frequent or long visits to their newborns in the NICU (Neonatal Intensive Care Unit). In such conditions, women often feel helpless and alienated. At the same time, women are now starting to vocalize their needs and to use all possible resources to change the situation, and maternity care providers are beginning to respond by changing their emotional style, as we will discuss in Chapter 5.

Women have to mobilize all kinds of the social, cognitive, informational and financial resources at their disposal in order to create personal trust and receive better care. For instance, most of our interlocutors planned their pregnancy and childbirth care, made multiple choices, acted strategically even within the institutionally set care trajectory, chose the place for their prenatal consultations, made choices about which childbirth training courses to take, defined their preferences about (un)desired medical procedures and looked for the best maternity hospital and care providers that would embody their ideas of "good care." After childbirth, they continue with the same strategy – they search for information, make careful choices of medical facilities and doctors to take care of their child and vary free services (under mandatory health insurance) with paid ones.

The social class position of those women who are ready to pay for individual obstetricians and midwives allows them to benefit from personalized relationships of trust with these practitioners. Such relationships often eliminate the discontinuity of care, uncertainty, and risks of emotional suffering that characterize "free" birth. In paid birth, women and providers create a closer and more prolonged contact – a kind of "chemistry" (attachment) with the chosen obstetrician or midwife (Temkina & Rivkin-Fish, 2020) that entails the ability to call and ask questions (Borozdina, 2016) and to discuss the birth plan. Having to resort to specialists might end that personal relationship and will certainly engage a patient into a very complicated set of logics and logistics, as described in the preceding chapter. Yet to avoid this discontinuity of care and its likely ensuing traumas, such providers involve a patient in their own inter-professional network of "proper" physicians who share the same notions and approach to "good care" – meaning humanistic care (see Davis-Floyd, 2018). This can be extremely important for women with a high probability of complications during pregnancy and childbirth.

Personalized relationships with maternity care practitioners also mean that women will entrust the decisions about their health to that person in a personalized, but still quite paternalistic, way. Affluent women who pay for such services are more interested in receiving "good care" (including emotional support) than in challenging the medicalization of their condition (Borozdina, 2016; Temkina, 2019; Temkina & Rivkin-Fish, 2020) or the authority of obstetricians. While many women in general are interested in natural birth (without artificial stimulation of labor and some other medical manipulations), they are more likely to rely on their chosen obstetrician's decisions rather than on their own personal opinions.

Many women combine pregnancy monitoring in public free-of-charge "women's consultations" (*zhenskaya konsul'tatsia*) with visits to private clinics for gaining more personal attention, more comfort and more control. A paid doctor is usually considered as *svoi* ("her own," the one whom she trusts) (see also Grødeland & Holmes, 2019). As explained in Chapter 3, while usually there are different obstetricians and facilities that provide care at different stages – from preconception to postpartum – the "paid" obstetrician is the one who can create the desired continuity of care (which is quite atypical in Russian maternity care). For instance, a woman can choose an obstetrician who will consult with her during pregnancy and attend her delivery; as 29-year-old Alia said: "*For the many questions that arose, I asked the doctor in the [free women's consultation]. And also asked the paid doctor with whom I planned to give birth. [It was important to me]* to *get a good, clear opinion from a knowledgeable person.*"

Women accept now that a "rightfully chosen" "doctor knows best." An obstetrician who is selected on the basis of a preliminary investigation of her/his reputation and with whom an emotional contact is established ceases to be a depersonalized actor of the unreliable State system of maternity care. "Establishing trust" means that the woman recognizes the authority and professionalism of the obstetrician, and through this recognition, indirectly controls the situation, while the obstetrician recognizes the patient as a person, and not just as an object of medical interventions. If earlier the mechanism of "bribe-blat" worked in this way, then under the consumerization and commercialization of maternity care, trust can be formed by choosing (and sometimes paying) for services. Such a project differs from simple "shopping around," as personalization constitutes the most important ground for trust. The most effective and rewarding personal relationships are described as having a special "spark." A "spark" is a metaphor for the strong intuition that the woman believes she may have when she feels trust in a particular practitioner – an obstetrician or a midwife – and that they are now connected in some special way. The childbearing woman is now ready to recognize that practitioner's authority and to delegate the management of childbirth, for which the practitioner takes leadership, personal and legal responsibility.

Thirty-one-year-old Marta, who carried out a thorough preliminary search to help her choose, describes her first meeting with her future obstetrician: "*When I came to my (future) doctor, she told me: 'Listen, you will listen to me carefully, and everything will be fine with you.'*" Marta continued by saying that this obstetrician might not support her initial plans, yet she preferred this obstetrician due to the "spark." She emphasized that the obstetrician herself would make the decisions. For a successful childbirth, as many interlocutors stated, the woman needs to obey the physician, follow her instructions and hope for the best.

> *You have to listen to what the doctor says. . . . The doctor will not give bad advice . . . listen and follow.*
>
> (interview with Alia, mother, age 29)

> *The main thing, as I understand it, is to obey the doctor, to trust.*
>
> (interview with Tatijana, mother, age 28)

After choosing providers, as is clear in these quotations, Russian women then tend to delegate control to them and identify them as trustworthy, reliable and efficient. As many interlocutors described, during labor and birth, "*the brain turns off, and you don't understand anything*" (interview with Emma, mother, age 27). "*And somehow it starts to work in some other direction . . . you already, as it were, do not make any decisions. . . . You forget to think about everything around you*" (interview with Inna, mother, age 34). Childbearing women believe that they cannot think and act rationally during labor and delivery, so they need reliable care provided by the health practitioners, who control what is going on. Women consciously take the position of obedient patients, trusting their obstetricians and delegating their agency to those obstetricians. Clearly, such women have fully internalized the principles of Russian paternalism (described in Chapter 3). They exercise their agency via their choice of hospital and practitioner(s), then surrender it completely during labor and birth.

However, some women report a more egalitarian "partnership" established with a maternity care provider. Agata, age 31, in comparing her experiences of her first and second births, describes how her relationships had changed from authoritarian (obstetrician took actions that were against her will) to partnership and dialogue:

> *I didn't have . . . that something is being done to me against my will [as happened during the first birth] . . . this time everything was so clear, it is clear why it was necessary. And the attitude of the doctor contributes*

> *to this. That is, when the obstetrician explains everything to you* [there is] *some kind of normal dialogue.*

Viktoria, age 28, continues:

> *We talked with [the doctor] for a very long time. . . . as if on an equal footing . . . It was such a partnership.*

Women appreciate providers' emotional labor as well, especially if they pay for service. Some interlocutors say that when paying, they expect and get more attention from providers:

> *They somehow warmly look there, smile, well, apparently, they understand that the person paid the money, and now they need to at least listen to her.*
>
> (interview with Nonna, mother, age 29)

> *[The privileged (paid) position creates] the feeling that I'm someone's daughter there. Everyone who participated in this process there, everyone with a smile, everyone is very kind, polite, pleasant.*
>
> (interview with Alia, mother, age 29)

Positive changes are not only visible in the commercial segment of care, although they are interrelated with its development. In State-funded ("free of charge") maternity care, we also observe notable changes both in women's demands and providers' behaviors. Both physical infrastructure, professionalism and emotional labor have notably improved compared to Soviet and early post Soviet times. Many women report satisfaction with the quality of care they receive. Such women write positive reviews on websites, express gratitude to the health providers and present them gifts regardless of whether they pay money officially or not. Here is an excerpt from our 2020 interview with Elvira, age 38:

Q: *Was this for free?*

Elvira: *Yes. There were very good conditions, I mean there is good food, everything is always clean, all of the cleaners, when they come, [called us nice names] like "bunnies", "sweeties" . . . I mean they are all positive, constantly making jokes, trying to make whatever good for us, and you can see that. . . . All are very friendly.*

These interlocutor descriptions of positive, warm care indicate that quite often, humanistically inclined medical personnel behave like quasi-mothers to these women. Nevertheless, the number of complaints keeps growing, both on websites and in letters written to official State bodies. Maternity care providers call this trend "patient extremism" and code such complaints as "unreasonable" and "consumerist," saying that it is impossible to satisfy such women in most State-funded facilities. Hence, we can see that these service-oriented women have created a new set of challenges for Russian maternity care. We will elaborate on this more in Chapter 5, where we will discuss how care providers cope with the changing natures of power relations and patients' demands. Here we present the perspectives of women who articulate their discontents.

Childbearing women's discontents with maternity care

In this section, we describe the growth of women's discontents and complaints, explain how these complaints are connected to women's expectations and analyze what in the Russian context of maternity care is fostering growing discontent.

The growth of complaints

Our data show an increase in the grievances and complaints of childbearing women. Maternity care providers in our empirical site, the Hospital, endlessly note that they are receiving more and more complaints, and this is a major concern for them, as we will further discuss in Chapter 5. The numerous complaints to different official bodies systematically create institutional and personal challenges to the Hospital's administrators and clinicians, as the complaints are followed up by State commissions' numerous inspections, fees and sanctions.

As the maternity care providers at the Hospital consider, they do their best for patients, and so they cannot understand the reasons for women's grievances, finding them unfair and explaining them away as caused by women's personal negative traits, stereotyping the patients who made the complaints as "aggressive" or "ignorant" (see Chapter 5). In fact, the significant growth of such complaints and attempts to prevent them or standardize their resolution preceded the interest of Hospital administration in sociological studies and our collaboration with them (see Chapter 2). They wondered what practices or communicational gaps resulted in these complaints.

According to a meta-ethnography of complaint analysis (Scott & Grant, 2018), patients worldwide complain about their dehumanization and objectification, the disrespectful ways in which they are treated by staff, their negative stereotyping, and providers who do not want to take responsibility for the results. Women say that during labor and birth, they are made to feel like inanimate objects in a "production line." Meanwhile, providers categorize those who complain or fight back as "bad patients," as egotistic, with low intelligence, childishness, dishonesty and/

or psychological maladjustment (ibid.). Women in the Hospital (as well as in the other Russian maternity facilities) make similar complaints and are stereotyped and judged by providers in similar ways. However, there are special organizational contexts of maternity care in Russia (Chapter 3) that cause particular kinds of dissatisfaction and misunderstandings, consequently leading to women's negative evaluations of their childbirth experiences.

As part of our fieldwork, we collected negative reviews on various websites about childbirth experiences in the Hospital. We also analyzed the more general, country-wide situation by looking at the postings on the Russian online campaign "violence-in-childbirth" *(nasilie-v-rodah)* involving different hospitals in different regions; we also refer to our interviews with women who received maternity care both in the Hospital and other maternity care facilities.

The mechanics of dissatisfaction: expectations vs. evaluations

As our research shows, complaints are embedded in a broad social context and a special temporality – women have expectations *before* the birth, which are generated by childbirth training courses, discussions with peers, websites (parental forums and social media) and care providers from different facilities. These expectations precede their experiences in the Hospital, which consequently are evaluated in comparison with their expectations. *Right after* childbirth, some women consider their birth experience to be positive simply because they ended up with a healthy baby. Yet *after leaving* the Hospital, mothers return to their social networks and actively discuss their labor and birth experiences, both online and in person. The comparisons and evaluations of others sometimes cause women to redefine and re-evaluate their own experiences as imperfect or negative. In some cases, public critical comments of women (expressed on websites or in written complaints) surprise Hospital providers – why did mothers express these complaints one year or more after delivery?

However, the most challenging complaints for providers are not those posted on websites as reviews or evaluations of the facility's or practitioners' work, but those that are sent to the State's bodies – *Rospotrebnadzor, Roszrdavnadzor*, regional and federal authorities, and in some most critical cases to the prosecutor's office or directly to the President (for more details on regulation by State bodies, see Chapter 3). Such officially submitted complaints by law must be processed by the hospital's administration and cause additional, laborious and time-consuming managerial and paperwork for physicians. Moreover, some complaints can provoke additional inspections by these controlling State bodies and, thus, interfere greatly with the regular work of the organization.

As we noted earlier, some women have relatively high expectations about how their pregnancies and births should go. Scholars claim that a complaint is an account of the violation of the patient's personal expectations for care (Lloyd-Bostock & Mulcahy, 1994; Scott & Grant, 2018). However, as our research demonstrates, both women and providers often consider expectations to be unrealistic. Sometimes patients and health practitioners in interviews and women on websites ironically say that these expectations look like "vanilla pictures" (a metaphor for high, unrealistic anticipations).

Textual analyses show that experiences in the Hospital are compared with attitudes formed by reviews on the internet written by peers or discussed with friends; ideas of "natural childbirth" on websites promoted by women, some attendants, midwives and doulas; a woman's own or her peer's childbirth experience in another hospital; and the image of the Hospital as a modern, high-tech institution with a very good reputation. As one of the users on the Littleone.com website (parental online forum) described:

> *I had chosen a maternity hospital, firstly, then a doctor . . . I had read articles and reviews about her, and I really liked her, and after talking to her, I decided to give birth with her . . . because I chose a doctor hoping that she would listen to me and my wishes. How naïve [I was].*
>
> (online forum, for more details on this and other such comments, see Appendix 5)

Another user compares two of her childbearing experiences to rank the Hospital:

> *It is no coincidence that the Hospital's rating is creeping downward. After reading the admiring reviews at the beginning of the year, I decided that I wanted to give birth only here. But, alas, my experience has not confirmed these enthusiastic reviews. I gave birth to my elder daughter few years ago in Maternity Hospital O. And comparing now, I can say that O. was better.*
>
> (online forum)

However, maternity hospitals are not flexible institutions, and they can only minimally adapt to such expectations, new ideas and needs shaped by the consumerization of patients' behavior and the emergence of the maternity services market. Thus, many women find that their expectations of "good care" are not met, even when they did everything they could to prepare. Yet obviously, establishing a good relationship with a care provider does not ensure that this practitioner will act as a woman wishes.

Mainstream trends in complaints

Among the main complaints in reviews on websites are organizational uncertainties, unreasonable medical interventions (e.g., induction of labor), (in)actions and neglect of clinicians to the course of labor (e.g., not conducting cesarean on time), contradictory recommendations, restrictions on free behavior in labor and *khamstvo* (rudeness). We argue that many complaints appear not as the result of the (in)actions of providers (as women often say) but are mostly due to the lack of recipients' understanding of what's going on. They notice the prevalence of managerial (bureaucratic logics), organizational failures and contradictions in the formal and informal rules regulating the field. Childbearing women and care providers have different interpretations of (in)actions and appropriate styles of behavior. Again, obstetricians believe that they do their best for their patients. They also understand (as the patients do not) that they have to maneuver among different norms and rules, instructions and limitations, among professional, market and bureaucratic logics. We will discuss the institutional challenges faced by clinicians from their perspectives in Chapter 5. In the following, we describe primary reasons for women's dissatisfaction with their hospital care.

(1) *Mistrust* is the primary reason for women's dissatisfaction, according to our findings. Many women initially believe that providers do not act in the interests of their patients. Women's evaluations of their childbearing experiences are rooted in their primary expectations, later comparisons with other birth stories, and their lay interpretations of the medical procedures applied to them during labor. Evaluations of birth experiences by care providers and receivers usually mismatch if women do not receive comprehensive information and explanations on the course of birth and treatment from their physicians; thus, women can interpret provider's (in)actions as incorrect and unprofessional. They may blame providers for not meeting their demands, for causing them harm and for acting in selfish interests (to save money, to enhance the statistics on cesarean birth, etc.). One woman claimed in retrospect (on a website) that her situation was wrongly defined, that her obstetrician acted according to his own comfort and convenience and that he cheated her out of the experience she desired and had been promised. In such cases, a woman feels herself as an object of deception and as a victim; she loses trust in maternity care providers, does not believe in the legitimacy of their actions and therefore complains.

(2) *Discontinuity of care* is the second structural reason for women's dissatisfaction. It manifests when women have to deal with multiple providers who have different approaches and give different recommendations; and when women face problems of communication and coordination during their routes in medical institutions. For example, just as a laboring woman gets used to her obstetrician and midwife, the shift can change and she will have to continue the labor with an entirely new group of practitioners.

Women share their experiences saying that labor had been going well, *"but when the shift began and the midwife changed, then it all [the negative experience] started"* (online forum). One shift, for example, was ready to wait and monitor the natural course of labor without intervention, but the next shift, which had changed in mid-labor, immediately started to augment labor with synthetic oxytocin (which causes the contractions to be longer, stronger and more painful, and is not needed in normal physiologic births, but can be beneficial in case of some complications of the process). The lack of communication between providers and women can lead to different understandings of the situation and the actions taken. This woman interpreted this labor augmentation as an unnecessary intervention that ruined her birth experience, whereas the providers saw it as a reasonable tactic. Women who have such experiences then draw conclusions about unreasonable clinical practices and poor coordination between shifts that caused harm to her or her newborn. This example illustrates that communication between shifts can be non-existent, to the great detriment of the patient. In addition, there is no clear way for a patient to call for the attention or assistance of the medical personnel; this lack can deepen her feeling of vulnerability and is often supplemented by helplessness and the inability to overcome organizational discoordination.

Let us give an example where a woman compares different styles of care and practices by different providers:

> *The wonderful midwife . . . helped during all stages and even after discharge, the nurses are wonderful – you could contact them at any time with questions about the baby's care and health. But, the terrible attitude of one nurse – rude and cynical, and some doctors at the postpartum, exhausted all my nerves.*
>
> (online forum)

(3, 4) *Inappropriate communication and emotional style* are the third and fourth major reasons for women's complaints. In the latter case, providers are blamed for not caring enough, or for practicing *khamstvo*. As previously noted, women who gave birth in Soviet or early post-Soviet periods often referred to obstetricians' and midwives' boorishness and neglect of their individual needs in a conveyer-like service, in which overloaded wards and ignorant, brusque, and overburdened personnel were common (Shhepanskaja, 1999; Rivkin-Fish, 2005). And now in the 2020s, our research reveals that women still face *khamstvo*. Aleksandra, age 30, said: "*Yes, they are boors. They yell, damn it, but they don't just yell, they discipline.*" Ariana, age 25, claimed,

> *The midwives were so angry, so conniving and insolent . . . and I asked her: "Well, what about the test results?". She snapped at me then: "How do I know, it's none of my business", and so on.*

As a consequence, dissatisfied patients feel themselves deceived and vulnerable, both emotionally (*bad, scared, powerless and hopeless*), socially (*feeling lonely, helpless, abandoned*) and physically (*feel painful, tired, discomfort*).

(5) *Lack of comfort* is the fifth major cause of the consumer complaints published online. Women complain about the conditions and the small size of birth rooms, low quality of food, uncomfortable beds and the rigid regime, which limits visitor access and restricts patients' abilities to move around within the Hospital. The following are quotes from the parental forum:

> *In a disposable shirt, which with each movement rises above the waist, lying for 3 hours is extremely uncomfortable. Until I asked for a sheet, no one thought to give one to me. Again, in Hospital O. it was more pleasant to lie on a normal bed . . . with normal sheets.*
>
> *The audibility is simply awful – from other birthplaces you can hear so much that it becomes scary long before your own delivery, there was a feeling as if others were giving birth with open doors, although this was not so.*
>
> *In the cafeteria, they feed products that are prohibited for breastfeeding . . . in each room there is a booklet with recommendations on the diet for breastfeeding, [in which] cucumbers are not allowed. And what do you think? They give me a cucumber for lunch, and this has happened many times.*
>
> *Relatives were not allowed to come, because this room was located on the territory of the maternity (delivery) ward. [I had to fight to get the things left for me at the reception.]*
>
> (online forum)

In sum, the Hospital is perceived by complaining women as a place of social isolation, lack of needed attention and emotional support, uncertain rules that change when the shift does, and complicated coordination, in which patients feel themselves vulnerable and helpless as they are shifted from provider to provider. In negative reviews, they claim that there are no or not enough conditions to meet their basic needs; that the administration and their practitioners are too inflexible; and that providers do not want to or cannot be sensitive to these needs. The contrasts between expectations and efforts to get "good care," and the care they actually receive, become negatively salient for them.

Nevertheless, we note once again that many women are satisfied with the care they receive in the Hospital, are thankful to the care providers who attended their births and plan to return for subsequent births. Here we concentrate only on those cases in which patients are not satisfied and express this publicly. We also leave aside situations with tragic outcomes. These situations call for special analysis that is beyond the scope of this book.

Now we turn to the recently emerged and widespread discourse on "violence in delivery," which includes articulations of practices of "obstetric aggression" that women faced during delivery, including intensive forms of those mentioned earlier.

The online campaign "nasilie-v-rodah" ("*violence in childbirth*")

In its most accessible form, women's dissatisfaction is represented in the public online campaign "for childbirth without violence" (vk.com/humanize_birth), placed at the Russian *VKontakte* social network (see data description in Appendix 6). The analysis of this data helps to delineate more broadly women's dissatisfactions in the field of contemporary maternity care. The moderators of this network explain that they aim to articulate the problem of violence in childbirth and defend the rights of women to seek humanized institutionalized childbirth, given that many women are subjected to obstetric aggression. Humiliation, trauma and pain are at the center of these women's stories from various Russian cities and maternity hospitals. Maternity care services in Russia are quite heterogeneous across regions and in the regional centers (Novkunskaya, 2020). However, some features of the state-funded, facility-based maternity care are common in most Russian hospitals (and also in some other post-Soviet societies, where women also participate in similar public campaigns). Women from different social contexts describe their suffering from various forms of obstetric violence, including rudeness, disrespect, incivility, neglect, deception and abusive treatment during birth.

Women want their childbirth to be the happiest event in their lives, but at a certain moment, for some women, "*The fairytale is over . . . Everything flew into the abyss. Needless to say, I left there dead, a woman and a mother with suicidal thoughts and prolonged postpartum depression*" (online post with the hashtag #nasilievrodah; for more details see Appendix 6).

Women talk about indifferent professionals who refuse to inform them, to answer their questions, to consider their needs and to take into account their fears and pain. Care providers take actions against women's will and put emotional and physical pressure on them in labor. Women say that they were shouted at, treated boorishly and accused of exaggerating and lying about their suffering: "*The doctor yelled that 'it cannot be painful', and I am a 'fool-pretender'*"(online post, #nasilievrodah).

Mothers describe being accused of not being able to fulfill their "main function" – to give birth and be a "good mother." A "bad mother" is a "potential killer" who harms the child's health:

> *The midwife yelled at me so that I would not howl, but breathe, like scolding a child, telling me what a disgusting mother I am. Doctors scared me that my child could be born an idiot!*
>
> (online post, #nasilievrodah)

As a result of such obstetric aggression, there is a withdrawal not only of agency as the ability to make and share decisions but also of the resources for the production of identity of a "responsible mother." Women write that they cannot speak, they are afraid to ask questions, feel helpless, do not understand what is happening to them, believe that they are being deceived and feel themselves as victims. They are objectified, reduced to their bodies, which are *tormented, torn, raped, trampled and broken*. Some women internalize these messages: they see themselves as "bad mothers," admit their inferiority and accuse themselves of wrong behavior:

> *It was a shame that I could not give birth, that I was a weakling, I was torturing a child. I hate myself, I am weak, not mature enough for motherhood!*
>
> (online post, #nasilievrodah)

By articulating their suffering on such online campaigns or resources, women try to make their voices heard ("the personal is political"). However, little institutional attention is given to this flashmob; women write mostly anonymously, and such online activities have a limited effect at the institutional level. However, it does manifest women's consciousness raising and publicizes their ideas about the need for the humanization of childbirth in Russia. While women have become more assertive as consumers and clients, within the medical field they have remained mostly silent and obedient as patients who feel that they cannot give voice to their pain. Interactions in maternity hospitals have become less paternalistic only to a limited extent, and complaints do not bring significant results and changes, though providers have become much more attentive to them and identify them as challenges for their professional practices.

Conclusion: the paradoxes of women's agency

Russian women, especially from the middle class, as assertive consumers, want to control their births at least enough to receive "good care" in maternity hospitals. For this purpose, they try to organize the best services they can afford, depending on their class position and access to resources. Childbearing women undertake detailed searches for information about hospitals and providers, identify what they want and do not want to face during pregnancy and delivery and articulate their own needs and expectations. Women try to achieve trust in personalized, often paid, relations with their primary care provider. However, such efforts are often not enough to guarantee "good care."

Acting as consumers, women seek empowerment through relationship, but frequently do not achieve it, as relationships in hospitals do not become egalitarian, they lack shared decision-making, and points of arrangements vanish with the coming of the new shift. The fairly recent market-orientation has led to a certain change in patient-provider interactions, but this shift does not radically change the emotional style of intra-hospital communication (more on that in Chapter 5) and does not actually challenge the paternalistic organization of Russia's maternity care system.

Scholars have shown that in different contexts, women have long struggled for recognition of their agency, and in some high-resource countries have indeed become more empowered in childbirth, which, though still highly medicalized, has also become more egalitarian, more humanistic and women-centered, more choice-oriented, and often provides continuity of care and a variety of options (Davis-Floyd, 2018; Davis-Floyd & Cheyney, 2019, 2022).

Women in Russia who want to acquire agency, make choices and ensure "good care" are now facilitated by both new attitudes toward motherhood and consumer-oriented behavior. Reformed maternity care is declared to be aimed at the improvement of the quality of care and improved conditions, especially in the commercial wards and private clinics. However, the changes in childbearing women's agency in Russia are not associated with collective actions or voice, or social movements and human rights, but mostly with individual efforts, resources and personalized negotiations. This only slightly changes the disposition of power and does not influence maternity care as a whole.

Many maternity care institutions remain to a large extent unfriendly to women, leaving them vulnerable and often unsatisfied with their childbirth experiences – unless they did manage to create trust via multiple negotiations with providers in advance, or were simply lucky to get the services they expected. Consumeristic relations in maternity care do not create childbearing women's collective empowerment. Rather, they create a contradiction: patients now behave individually as active consumers, and their demands for "good care" increase, but in general, care providers are unable to fully satisfy women's demands, as they do not have enough autonomy to humanize care and often are not willing to soften their emotional style. Providers in some cases do personalize their relationships with patients and negotiate care, but do not intend to share decision-making. This kind of relationship seems fine with all those women who, once they have exercised their agency by choosing their provider and their hospital, passively submit themselves to whatever the provider decides. Thus, women's agency is embedded in individual efforts to achieve "good care" via the choices they make, while, paradoxically, childbearing women continue to endow obstetricians with paternalist power, expecting that they will solve any problem. This can lead to positive results, or, conversely, to complaints, if expectations are not met, especially when the treatment is overtly rude and abusive.

We have noted the increase in such complaints, in which women, as elsewhere worldwide, describe their objectification and humiliation. However, special problems characterize Russian maternity care, associated with poor coordination and the absence of continuity of care. In hospitals, providers must constantly deal with organizational uncertainty and contradictory rules, which systematically lead to misunderstandings, such as when women suspect providers of acting in their own interests and not in those of their patients. Practitioners are not used to providing comprehensive explanations; thus, women often do not understand what is happening and what are the reasons for care providers' actions. As a result, they blame physicians and midwives for irrelevance, mistakes, neglect and are especially horrified by *khamstvo* – the rude emotional style that is still in use – this is precisely what most women seek to avoid during labor and birth. Thus, women are still coming home from maternity hospitals with "horror stories," which circulate online as shared negative evaluations of maternity care.

Although maternity care providers evaluate negative reviews or complaints to various State bodies as "irrelevant" and "unfair," such complaints provide opportunities for women to make their voices heard. They can use the internet or formal letters to government bodies to express their criticisms. Sometimes women try to find their own ways to solve or avoid potential problems: to change a provider or hospital, to involve third parties and intermediaries or to use informal agreements, but these individual actions do not improve the overall situation. Having focused on childbearing women in this chapter, in the next we turn to care providers' positions and perspectives on the issues raised herein.

References

Avdeeva, A. (2020). *Natural Parenting in Contemporary Russia: When 'Nature' Meets Kinship*. Doctoral thesis, University of Helsinki. Available at: https://helda.helsinki.fi/handle/10138/316260 (Accessed 03.04.2021).

Borozdina, E. (2016). Zabota v rodovspomozhenii: vygody i izderzhki professionalov [Professional care in maternity hospitals: Benefits and challenges]. *Zhurnal Issledovaniy Sotsial'noy Politiki [The Journal of Social Policy Studies]*, 14(4), 479–92.

Cook, L. J. (2017). Constraints on universal health care in the Russian federation: Inequality, informality and the failures of mandatory health insurance reforms. In Y. Ilcheong (Ed.), *Towards Universal Health Care in Emerging Economies* (pp. 269–296). London: Palgrave Macmillan.

Davis-Floyd, R. E. (2001). The technocratic, humanistic, and holistic paradigms of childbirth. *International Journal of Gynecology & Obstetrics*, 75(S5).

Davis-Floyd, R. E. (2003). *Birth as American Rite of Passage* (2nd ed.). Berkeley: University of California Press.

Davis-Floyd, R. E. (2018). Open and closed knowledge systems, the 4 stages of cognition, and the cultural management of birth. *Frontiers in Sociology*, 3(23). https://doi.org/10.3389/fsoc2018.2018.0023.

Davis-Floyd, R. E., & Cheyney, M. (2019). *Birth in Eight Cultures*. Long Grove, IL: Waveland Press.

Davis-Floyd, R. E., & Cheyney, M. (2022). *Birth as an American Rite of Passage* (3rd ed.). Abingdon, Oxon: Routledge.

Godovannaya, M., & Temkina, A. (2017). 'Mat ty navechno, no i khudozhnitsa – vsegda': tvorchestvo v usloviyakh intensivno-rasshirennogo materinstva ['You are a mother forever, but an artist for good, as well': Creative work in the context of intensive-extensive mothering]. *Laboratorium: Russian Review of Social Research*, 9(1), 30–61 (In Russian).

Grødeland, Å. B., & Holmes, L. (2019). Nash chelovek. *Global Informality Project.* Available at: www.in-formality.com/wiki/index.php?title=Nash_chelovek_(Russia_and_FSU).

Hays, Sh. (1996). *The Cultural Contradictions of Motherhood.* New Haven: Yale University Press.

Korotkikh, E., & Popova, V. (2017). Platnye rody: ozhidaniya patsientok i osobennosti vzaimodeystviya s akusherkoy' [Paid childbirth: Patients' expectations and relationships with a Midwifes]. In E. Borozdina & A. Temkina (Eds.), *Menyayushcheesya rodovspomozhenie: vzglyad akusherok i sotsiologov* [*Changes in Childbirth: Midwifery and Sociological Perspectives*] (pp. 24–30). Preprint collection. St. Petersburg: European University at St Petersburg Press (In Russian).

Liese, K., Davis-Floyd, R., Stewart, K., & Cheyney, M. (2021). Obstetric iatrogenesis in the United States: The spectrum of disrespect, violence, and abuse. *Anthropology & Medicine*, 28(2), 188–204. https://doi.org/10.1080/13648470.2021.1938510.

Lloyd-Bostock, S., & Mulcahy, L. (1994). The social psychology of making and responding to hospital complaints: An account model of complaint processes. *Law & Policy*, 16, 123–147.

Novkunskaya, A. (2020). Some symptoms of neoliberalisation in the institutional arrangement of maternity services in Russia. In J. Gabe, M. Cardano, & A. Genova (Eds.), *Health and Illness in the Neoliberal Era in Europe* (pp. 177–193). Bingley: Emerald Publishing Limited. https://doi.org/10.1108/978-1-83909-119-320201010.

Novkunskaya, A., Litvina, D., & Temkina, A. (2020). Khamstvo (USSR, Russia). *Global Informality Project.* Available at: https://www.in-formality.com/wiki/index.php?title=Khamstvo_(USSR,_Russia) (Accessed 19.07.22).

Radzinsky, V. E. (2011). *Akusherskaja agressija* [*Obstetric Aggression*]. Moscow; Status Praesens.

Rivkin-Fish, M. (2005). *Women's Health in Post-Soviet Russia: The Politics of Intervention.* Bloomington: Indiana University Press.

Sadler, M., Santos, M. J., Ruiz-Berdún, D., Rojas, G. L., Skoko, E., Gillen, P., & Clausen, J. A. (2016). Moving beyond disrespect and abuse: Addressing the structural dimensions of obstetric violence. *Reproductive Health Matters*, 24(47), 47–55. https://doi.org/10.1016/j.rhm.2016.04.002.

Scott, D., & Grant, S. (2018). A meta-ethnography of the facilitators and barriers to successful implementation of patient complaints processes in health-care settings. *Health Expect*, 21, 508–517.

Shhepanskaja, T. B. (1999). Mifologija social'nyh institutov: rodovspomozhenie [The mythology of social institutions: Maternity care]. *Mifologija i povsednevnost'* [*Mythology and Everyday Life*], 3, 389–423 (In Russian).

Stepurko, T., Pavlova, M., Gryga, I., & Groot, W. (2013). Informal payments for health care services–corruption or gratitude? A study on public attitudes, perceptions and opinions in six Central and Eastern European countries. *Communist and Post-Communist Studies*, 46(4), 419–431.

Temkina, A. (2017). «Jekonomika doverija» v platnom segmente rodovspomozhenija: gorodskaja obrazovannaja zhenshhina kak potrebitel' i pacientka ['The economy of trust' in the paid segment of obstetrics: An educated urban woman as a consumer and a patient]. *Jekonomicheskaja sociologija [Economic Sociology]*, 18(3), 14–53 (In Russian).

Temkina, A. (2018). Budushchaya mat kak issledovatel: strategii organizatsii platnykh rodov v rossiyskom krupnom gorode [Mother-to-be as a field researcher: The strategies of private obstetrics provision in Urban Russia]. *Antropologicheskij forum [Anthropological Forum]*, 37, 198–230. http://anthropologie.kunstkamera.ru/fi%20les/ (In Russian).

Temkina, A. (2019). 'Childbirth is not a car rental': Mothers and obstetricians negotiating consumer service in Russian commercial maternity care. *Critical Public Health*, 30(5), 521–532. https://doi.org/10.1080/09581596.2019.1626004.

Temkina, A., Litvina, D., & Novkunskaya, A. (2021). Emotional styles in Russian maternity hospitals: Juggling between *khamstvo* and smiling. *Emotions and Society*, 3(1), 95–113. https://doi.org/10.1332/263169021X16143466495272.

Temkina, A., & Rivkin-Fish, M. (2020). Creating health care consumers: The negotiation of un/official payments, power and trust in Russian maternity care. *Social Theory & Health*, 18, 340–357. https://doi.org/10.1057/s41285-019-00110-3.

Utrata, J. (2015). *Women without Men: Single Mothers and Family Changes in the New Russia*. Ithaca, NY: Cornell University Press.

Chapter 5

Providers negotiating multifaceted "good care"

The positions of medical providers in Russian maternity care are complex and ambiguous. Like other professional groups around the world, this profession is undergoing significant changes due to the influences of marketization and new managerial requirements (Scott et al., 2000; Freidson, 2001; Saks, 2015). Russian health and maternity care providers' positions are also shaped by the legacy of the Soviet organizational and cultural traits. As a result, a particular hybrid system of conflicting rules and requirements emerges, and ideas and practices of "good care" become confusing.

In previous chapters, we described the multiple inconsistencies and challenges that shape the ways in which maternity care is provided in Russia. On the one hand, maternity care providers still considerably depend on the State's direct regulation and control much more than on autonomous professional self-regulation: multiple bureaucratic requirements rigidly frame the rules in organizational settings and the working conditions of physicians, nurses and midwives (see Chapter 3). On the other hand, the emerging market of healthcare as well as changes in patients' expectations (see Chapter 4) influence the new ideals and practices of "good care."

In this chapter, we explain how "good care" became a multifaceted configuration of ideals and practices that are formulated on different levels and by different agents in maternity care – maternity care recipients, practitioners and the State. Moreover, the neoliberal policies of recent years create new spaces for some professional groups to offer their own notions and practices of "good care" in maternity hospitals – these are independent (mostly semi-legal) midwives, doulas,[1] commercial breastfeeding consultants and perinatal psychologists. Our research demonstrates that obstetricians, neonatologists and other physicians have to perform multiple roles (acting as clinicians, service providers, State bureaucrats) and apply various techniques (including *manual management* and increasing volumes of emotional labor) to cope with the inconsistencies and challenges that they face in their daily professional lives.

We begin this chapter with an analysis of multifaceted notions of "good care," then proceed with the analysis of multiple roles that maternity care

DOI: 10.4324/9781003139539-5

practitioners have to fulfill in order to meet new expectations and demands. In the second section, we describe the strategies and tools that maternity care providers use to meet these challenges and conflicting requirements by systematic "manual management." In the third section, we analyze "emotional labor" (in terms of Hochschild, 1983), which has to be done in order to meet multiple and various patient demands and to prevent complaints from consumer-oriented patients. In the end, we come to the conclusion that the professional groups of obstetricians, nurses and hospital midwives, who are socially considered to be in a powerful position, find themselves under overall control and are indeed limited in their possibilities to provide "good care."

We need to re-emphasize that maternity care in Russia is highly medicalized and that maternity hospitals (especially Level 3 hospital like our empirical site) have numerous departments and specialists involved in care provision: obstetricians, pediatricians, neonatologists, anesthesiologists, ultrasound specialists, surgeons, nurses, midwives, etc. Moreover, in complex clinical situations, narrower specialists join the team – geneticists, cardiologists, neuro-/cardiac surgeons, hematologists. In this section, we will talk about the perspectives and positions of maternity care providers – meaning all those who work in our field site (although we should mention that many of our arguments could be extrapolated to other medical settings in Russia). Although medical professionals of different specializations obviously have different professional cultures and positions, they follow similar institutional rules and face the same requirements and expectations from patients and the State. In other words, as *agents in the maternity care field*, they act in similar ways. Therefore, we mostly will universally refer to all medical professionals in this field as "practitioners" or "providers," sometimes without specification. When it is important to differentiate between different professional groups, we will make a relevant clarification.

Multifaceted maternity "good care": new actors and provider roles

What does it mean for practitioners to provide "good care" when they have so many referents – the State, their patients, the market, their professional community? Ideals and practices of "good care" are historically and culturally framed. Expectations toward maternity care practitioners are multicontextual – they have to perform multiple roles, including roles for which they are not fully prepared and qualified. This section addresses these issues, after first describing the current field of maternity care as comprised of multiple social actors, who bring different, and in some cases, conflicting ideas about "good care." Secondly, we turn to the analysis of the social roles that providers are to accomplish in order to fit multifaceted expectations and norms of "good" maternity care.

"Good care" as negotiated by different actors

In the frame of the structural-functional approach (and in medical practice as well), it is considered that both physicians and patients are accomplishing *normative* social roles set by institutional expectations and systems of social control (Parsons, 2013 [1951]). These roles are designed to maintain social order and assume that a physician is an expert in diagnosing and curing, while a patient's task is to cooperate. In such a model, physicians, as professionals, have a monopoly on expertise and knowledge and manage medical interactions on their own. Their role is narrow, functionally specific – limited to a specific field of medicine, and also affectively neutral (Ibid.).

The role of a patient in this approach is also functionally specific; it is expected that patients just obey and follow instructions. More than 70 years after Parsons' (1951) descriptions of healthcare roles, many obstetricians and other practitioners still expect this obedience from childbearing women in Russian maternity care. However, under the influence of globalization, consumerization and availability of information, patients worldwide no longer unconditionally trust and obey medical providers, who are not impartial experts to them anymore (Freidson, 1970). Patients worldwide are "shopping," comparing options and choosing a provider and treatment that suits their expectations of appropriate care (Lupton, 1997; Temkina, 2019). Patients – and especially childbearing women – are taking an increasingly active position and use the given options to make the best choices they can (Fotaki, 2013, 2014; Gabe et al., 2015). In Russia, the latest State policies and growing marketization support them in this endeavor (Chapter 4).

In the normative model, the State works as a frame – it provides appropriate conditions for "good care," which is exercised by medical professionals as the main experts and most powerful actors in this field. However, in Russia, the State was and still is the central actor in care provision, though the role of the commercial sector is growing and significantly changing the standards of "good care." The State – through healthcare policies and regulative standards for medical care and control – creates and shapes ideas and practices of "good care." In this post-Soviet bureaucratic-managerial logic, medical (including maternity) care provision is regulated by strict rules and orders, which make medical providers to a large extent accountable to the State and obedient to its requirements.

State control over medical professionals is designed in a bureaucratic way – via filling out a lot of documentation that consists of all sorts of information that is unnecessary in clinical practice, but makes sure that the organization fulfills institutional requirements (where to spend money, which medications to buy and when, etc.) and quantitative indicators of quality (infant and maternal mortality, amount of births, abortions, cesarean birth, etc.). Therefore, medical providers have to have "good indicators" (even if control over them is not in their power or conflicts with their clinical approach) in order to fit the criteria.

Established clinical, financial and organizational formal requirements and norms are formulated and controlled by various State bodies and others (see Chapter 3). They are numerous, sometimes contradictory, and tend to lag behind the contemporary situation in medicine in general (and the given organization in particular). Here is an example – a field note about a midwife who listed numerous controlling bodies that regularly monitor the Hospital and its documentation:

> *Alla Nikolaevna describes [different forms of regular] control – what regulatory systems exist and shape the work of the Hospital:*
>
> 1. *Rospotrebnadzor*
> 2. *Sanitary-epidemic norms*
> 3. *Orders issued by the Ministry of Health*
> 4. *The State standards and algorithms for performing manipulations*
> 5. *If there are no State standards, then organization makes up its own, approved by a special commission*
>
> (field notes, conversation with Alla Nikolaevna, chief midwife)

Thus, maternity care providers mostly act as State employees who carry out the State's notions of "good care" and introduce them into practice. However, these standards of care are undergoing change, and recently have become smoother under the globalization of evidence-based knowledge and marketization, in comparison with the more rigid Soviet approach. While in Soviet times, babies and mothers were separated, breastfeeding was limited, and partners were not allowed to come into the closed and opaque (non-transparent) maternity hospitals, in the new order of the Ministry of Health № 1130n (issued on the 12th of November 2020), as well as the previous one (№ 572n issued in 2012), the State body noted that:

> in obstetric hospitals, family-oriented (with a partner) childbirth is recommended . . . in the delivery room, in the absence of contraindications, it is recommended to ensure the earliest first attachment of the baby to the breast (no later than within 1.5–2 hours) after birth lasting at least 30 minutes and breastfeeding support. . . . In the postnatal departments, the joint stay of mother and newborn is recommended, as well as free access of family members to a woman and a child.
>
> (Ministry of Health, 2020)

As previously described, maternity care receivers have become more service-oriented, create their own expectations and demand new approaches to be practiced (see Chapter 4). In recent years, issues of communication with patients are being discussed at Russian medical conferences, and new professional standards are being set in some organizations and fields – especially in the most commercialized sectors, though not exclusively. Comfort, both physical and emotional, the humanization of childbirth, and more trusting, personalized relationships between maternity care providers and receivers have gradually become tangible requirements for practitioners. Obstetricians and midwives are gradually changing their approaches to childbirth, and some State recommendations correspond with these changes. However, providers are still limited in their possibilities to implement them full-scale.

Some midwives introducing and practicing new approaches fill in the niche of commercialized and more personalized care (Borozdina, 2016). Formally, they can work in Russian maternity care only as obstetricians' assistants; however, some midwives create niches for relatively autonomous care and now are struggling for institutional changes (Borozdina & Novkunskaya, 2020; see also Chapter 6). As some previous studies show (Borozdina, 2014; Borozdina & Novkunskaya, 2020) maternity care providers can initiate ground-level changes via introducing new, more women-oriented approaches and even via creating some spaces for midwifery autonomy (we will introduce some of the cases in Chapter 6). However, these cases contribute more to the empowerment of midwives than to enhancing women's participation in decision-making and empowerment.

The growing market of maternity care services influences State's "good care" ideals and also brings in more competitiveness by allowing new actors (such as doulas, independent midwives, breastfeeding consultants, perinatal psychologists, and even lawyers (Ozhiganova, 2020)) to enter hospitals and by providing new services (private birth rooms, the presence of partners during labor and delivery, "soft" birthing techniques). In such competition, "good care" has become a less coherent concept – encroach into the field of maternity care and, consequently, introduce new, sometimes alternative, ideals. These new actors can accomplish different tasks in maternity care: to defend patient rights and ensure that patients' expectations are fulfilled, to act as mediators between care receivers and care providers and to provide emotional and social support (Ozhiganova & Molodtsova, 2020). Doulas in particular reduce hospital midwives' workloads (do massage, bring water, "hold by hand") and can negotiate patient needs with obstetricians and other hospital staff, in some cases advocating and protecting women from overmedicalization. Though the legal position of doulas and independent midwives is uncertain, childbearing women often trust them and perceive them as a shield between themselves and standardized State-funded maternity care.

The multiplicity of social actors participating in care provision changes the landscape of maternity care, as they offer a more diverse palette of birthing and caring options, and higher and more personalized standards of "good care." At the same time, they are being accused by institutionalized medical providers of imbuing patients with mistrust of their own ("old") versions of "good care," formulating unrealistic expectations and gaining profit, along with having almost no legal responsibilities. These new agents and new practices are not always easy to replicate and to fit into the institutional order. Thus, institutionalized maternity care providers – obstetricians, other physicians and midwives practicing in medical settings – often respond negatively to these new actors and treat them in unfriendly ways. They argue that a multiplicity of different maternity care providers causes amplification of institutional inconsistencies – in particular, through the emergence of additional recommendations that in some cases contradict their own and appear unsuitable for a hospital. For example, some doulas advise waiting for labor to start on its own, and to allow women to adopt any positions they choose during labor, whereas local hospital staff members want to speed up the labor process and limit movement during labor – or there is no equipment in the hospital that facilitates upright positions.

Obstetricians and hospital midwives emphasize the absence of doulas' and independent midwives' legal responsibility. This is how a hospital midwife articulated this position in a public discussion with a psychologist: *"I refuse to perceive people who do not work in healthcare as helping specialists. There must work people who are somehow responsible for the result!"* (field notes). While obstetricians and hospital midwives understand maternity care primarily as responsibility for the clinical result (absence of negative medical consequences for mother and newborn), the growing segment of commercial "caring specialists," such as doulas and independent midwives, sees care as not exclusively clinical, but more holistically (Davis-Floyd, 2001, 2018; Davis-Floyd & Cheyney, 2022). In addition, the internet makes international medical publications available to the avant-garde of critically thinking Russian maternity care providers who are trying to find legal and organizational ways to bring the best practices and standards of care into Russian institutions (more on that in Chapter 6). These international "best practices" comprise another facet of the complex "good care" concept. The emerging competition between differing notions of "good care" brings new requirements for providers, especially the ones in the system of State-funded healthcare. Our research shows that maternity care providers have to extend their roles beyond their normative clinical ones and develop certain coping techniques as responses to the changing conditions and in order to provide "good care."

Expanding the role: the multiple tasks of hospital maternity care providers

Nowadays, physicians in maternity hospitals must widen their repertoire of roles to fulfill their own professional ideals and norms concerning the best ways in which childbirth should be managed. We will show how they have to act like State bureaucrats, effective managers, service workers, psychologists and many others. They do not perceive these tasks as "authentic" to their profession(s), but as practices they have to perform because there are no other agents in the field who could do this (or they are insufficient). These non-medical tasks are framed by those multifaceted "good care" ideals that pose expectations and requirements to primary maternity care providers. Therefore, they must learn tasks that they would prefer to delegate, as these tasks appear to be very resource intensive. Let us provide some examples.

Obstetricians and midwives nowadays manage increasing numbers of institutional inconsistences as parts of their working routines. Providers, especially in administrative positions, work as *coordinators* and *effective managers*, whose tasks are to coordinate the medical work of the Hospital or its unit, and to calculate budgetary flows and balance between service costs and revenues. The following field note, taken during the observation of the report on the work of the surgical department, illustrates the topicality of this role:

> *Oleg Borisovich [director of the Hospital] asks a question: "Do you [the surgical department] fit into the financing – in the incoming money via Federal quotas, Mandatory health insurance and combined sources? How much money has the [surgical] department earned? You have to be aware: do you cover your payroll or do we [the Hospital administration] subsidize you?"*
>
> *The head of the surgical department: "We would like to be subsidized, but we earn for ourselves."*
>
> (field notes)

In this example, the need to bargain between economic efficiency and clinical work brings new logic into the work of a surgeon, who is expected to increase the workload of his department in order to increase the funding. In this way, the market logic of regulation subordinates professional logic. As our data show, the role of an effective manager concerns not only those physicians and midwives who conduct administrative in addition to clinical work. The following quote from an interview with a midwife from the maternity department of the Hospital confirms the general concerns of providers around the economic aspect of maternity care provision:

> *Well, we have now become such people who can earn their own salaries and [some] would like to earn more, and accordingly, well . . . I don't know, in my opinion, this is wrong. Therefore, it turns out that we have to earn, earn, earn money.*
>
> (interview with Anzhelika, midwife)

This concern over the financial stability of maternity care is reinforced by the recent neoliberal policies and causes the need to routinely calculate the budget, minimize the use of consumables and invent new ways to earn money (via the introduction of paid services) to compete for patients. Maternity care providers appear to be personally involved in the management of the work in the Hospital; instead of thinking only about the clinical conditions of their patients, they have to perform roles that they haven't been prepared for, do calculations that they are unsure about:

> *We start a [new] clinical record [for the same patient and put there] a new nosology so that they will be paid somehow. Tariffs are greatly reduced. . . . There is less than half a million rubles [the quota for a premature child under 1500 grams]. . . . [But in fact] the costs are calculated in millions for such a child. Therefore, we (who are caring for premature babies) are always State-funded. . . . We think that when we have different clinical records, it helps to increase the payout from it. But I'm not an economist and I don't even know if it works or not.*
>
> (field notes, interview with head of department)

This physician is saying that she thinks that if they have multiple clinical records for the same patient, the State would cover each one with more money, compared to the payments they would get if they continued the same medical record. But in fact, she doesn't know whether this works or not, nor how the money is distributed by the State. She cannot do anything else for these patients – caring for premature babies will always be covered by the State (due to its high costs), and there is no other source from which she can get money.

Physicians of different specializations working in the Hospital are unfamiliar with economic processes and have to constantly consider *effectiveness* in terms of budget and quantitative indicators, while they understand that some clinical cases (such as caring for premature babies) will always be financially costly. Along with that, providers are expected to be client- and service-oriented, which makes many of them feel like they are *service providers* who are "selling" themselves, which lowers their professional status:

> *So we, in general, are ready to introduce pregnancy monitoring as a paid-for service, which we did not do before at all. So, well, in general we have come to this need because life is harsh, we are moving from the category of "help" to the category of "services." Regrettable as it may sound, in order to sell yourself, you need to do something. You have to change a bit somehow. You need to learn and somehow control yourself, learn to smile, to address the patient. And somehow slightly change your mind.*
>
> (interview with Alla Nikolaevna, chief midwife)

This new style of communication challenges practitioners' roles and authority, as one anesthesiologist complains: "*Some already perceive medicine as a service system*," and adds with irony: "*Should we smile to all of them then?*" (field notes). Maternity care providers say that it is not easy to get used to functioning as a "service worker" and to do the things that are not exactly "medical," but include actions aimed at the physical and emotional comfort of service-oriented patients.

Other non-clinical tasks derive from the need to be competent in legal and law-enforcement issues, as the field of childbirth is becoming more and more politicized and charged with legal proceedings. Providers have to learn legal requirements in order to protect themselves from patients' complaints and legal claims, which are increasing in relation to maternity care. They also should know legal norms in order to avoid possible sanctions and fines from controlling bodies. Many medical conferences regularly introduce "legal sections" to educate physicians and nurses (of various specializations) about how to protect themselves. Maternity care providers try to self-educate, although they still find these issues to be extremely complicated when they face problems to which they have no idea how to react. The following quotation from a conversation with a head of department shows such an embarrassment:

> *We are unprotected from anyone. If a mom wants to take the baby, should I give it? I don't know! We are not being taught what we should do. If a mom wants to change a physician, what should I do? I don't know. The local lawyer is incompetent. This lawyer office is oriented at procurements and contracts. No one is going to defend us in court . . . We open the Civil Code ourselves. Can a mom be responsible for a child if she is fifteen? I don't know, neither does the lawyer.*
>
> (field notes, interview with Valentina, head of department)

Both managerial and market logics exacerbate the necessity for maternity care providers to accomplish the tasks of a lawyer. On the one hand, they are to know all the standards and orders regulating maternity care provision. On the other, they face new patient expectations and demands, which can be in conflict with the formal rules, but in turn can trigger legal action. Thus, in order to accomplish professional work and avoid getting patient complaints, midwives, nurses, obstetricians, neonatologists and other practitioners have recently begun to act as *psychologists* – attentive to women's emotions, especially the feelings of those who have complicated clinical conditions or reproductive loss, which sometimes can take hours (in addition to their clinical work). Professional psychologists are present at the Hospital, but in insufficient numbers, and not all physicians know that psychologists are available and helpful (nor do childbearing women). A midwife of a prenatal ward describes this kind of work as an intrinsic part of her professional competence and role:

> *And if a woman at 30 weeks [of gestation] feels that her water is broken, she generally has a panic, [she worries] what will happen to her, she does not know whether her child will survive. That is, they think*

> *of what will happen to them, [if] such a misfortune has happened, and whether everything would get better – [in these cases] psychological help to women is also very important: conversations, talking. From time to time, almost all midwives know how to do it,* they *know how to do it.*
>
> (interview with Anna Alekseevna, midwife)

Maternity care providers speak a great deal about their "psychological" tasks as a part of their new professional duties, while they carry out emotional labor as practical experiences and intuitive decisions, rather than based on professional training and education. This kind of work regards not only midwives and nurses, who are considered to comprise the "caring professions" and are normatively expected to emotionally support women. As our data show, obstetricians and even the Hospital's administration articulate the necessity to work as "psychologists"; here is how one of the heads of department described it during an interview: *"They [women] are very unhappy. They often cry, just cry, here. They consider themselves very unhappy . . . Yes, we ourselves have already become psychotherapists"* (interview with Mila, head of department). She says that it is very important to speak to women, carefully explain their health condition and try to calm them down by listening and addressing their problems. But, according to her, most maternity care providers are not ready for such work, as there is no special training for it, and consequently, more experienced, senior physicians have to be left with this burden. However, many practitioners consider that it is very important to support women:

> *It happens that in the middle of the night a woman [at inpatient service] can go out and cry. You need to take her in the middle of the night, bring her, talk to her, calm her down. . . . I myself have had this . . . when a woman at three o'clock in the morning walked and sobbed. We examined her problem, sat down and talked.*
>
> (interview with Mila, head of department)

Providers have to care, to personally and emotionally support their patients, especially those in complicated and painful situations. The volume of emotional labor as an important component of "good care" increases and becomes an integral part of their professional work. We will address different tools of emotional labor later on in this chapter.

Such extra labor and extra care are not presupposed by the working duties, nor supported by institutional conditions. These skills are not learned in professional medical training, nor included in formal regulations and rules. These new maternity care providers' roles are mostly invisible, though participants in medical encounters are aware of them; these roles create an additional burden but have become an immanent part of the Russian maternity care landscape, constituting what we are terming the manual management of maternity care. This changing understanding of maternity care creates new challenges to providers' practice. They have to be aware of official requirements and standards, and financial restrictions; they have to be sensitive to women's growing expectations and demands under competition with new actors in the field and to balance between the formal rules and actual conditions of their work. In order to manage this multiplicity of new roles, providers apply and elaborate various tools, among which the main (and most systematic) tools, as we have observed in our field site, are *manual management* and *emotional labor*, which the following sections will address in detail.

Maternity care providers' manual management: handling multiple inconsistencies

Now we turn to answering the question of how maternity care providers routinely cope with contradictory demands and consequent challenges in their organizational settings. In order to maintain institutional order, they have to be personally involved in the micro- and macro-management of the Hospital work on different levels. Practitioners (physicians, nurses and midwives), especially those in administrative positions, become "communicators," personally connecting different care providers and receivers, specialists, departments, institutions, equipment, and resources to maintain workable conditions. As a result, not only do official standards and norms regulate the provision of care but also personified and informal interactions. This mostly invisible layer of their work constitutes the foundation of care provision, though this care is far from professional ideals.

Healthcare providers have been previously conceptualized as "street-level bureaucrats" or "frontline workers, as they simultaneously face severe workloads, experience conflicting demands from policy rules, their client's needs, their professional codes, and their own personal values" (Tummers et al., 2015, p. 1099). Starting from the classic work of Michael Lipsky (1980), social scientists have investigated different coping strategies elaborated by street-level bureaucrats in order to manage these practical dilemmas arising from the very nature of public services provision. Though there are multiple dimensions in which these coping strategies are developed by healthcare providers, including behavioral and cognitive dimensions (Tummers et al., 2015), in this section of the chapter, we aim to describe in detail those regarding the coordination of service provision that affects it at the organizational (not only individual) level. In particular, we will demonstrate how rule bending and breaking, and using personal resources help clients as some of the most widespread coping strategies for the frontline working contexts (ibid.) emerge and become integral parts of the Hospital's organizational order.

As shown in Chapters 3 and 4, systematic discontinuities in maternity care and inconsistencies among rules provoke challenges for the work of providers. On the one hand, these challenges come from the rigid State regulation, as controlling bodies regularly carry out inspections, and their sanctions are impossible to avoid: *"fines are inevitable, just accept it"* (field notes). On the other, the expectations of consumer-oriented clients grow and, not being met in all cases, cause an increase in the number of complaints, which, in turn, can trigger additional inspections by the State controlling bodies, and more sanctions can follow.

Under rigid, formal and hierarchical control, maternity care providers have to negotiate and coordinate their work informally when clinical necessity does not follow certain official rules, or rules do not exist, or are not updated, or contradict each other. In order to sustain the Hospital's organizational order, practitioners have had to implement many additional invisible coordinations and emotional labors. Here we analyze informal horizontal negotiations as one kind of coping strategy, accomplished personally by providers, which we call *manual management (ruchnoe upravlenie)*. In other words, maternity care providers have to negotiate with each other in order to solve numerous routine and urgent problems when official rules are unhelpful or contradictory. This invisible (to outsiders) work is aimed at navigating patients through organizational inconsistencies and, as a consequence, makes practitioners overloaded with duties and responsibilities, and also vulnerable.

In speaking about manual management, we refer to the term "manual control" used by scholars in their analyses of vertical power in the contemporary authoritarian regime in Russia, as these terms have both similarities and differences. "Manual control" (sometimes in Russian these terms refer to the same phenomenon – *ruchnoe upravlenie*; see, e.g., Monaghan, 2012) in political science refers to personal senior management of the electoral system (first of all, by the President and his team), federal reforms and the media (Petrov et al., 2010, 2014; Schenk, 2013). This term identifies the system in which Russia's "ruling elite relies on manual control, or personal intervention in the policy process" as a strategy to maintain political power (Petrov et al., 2010, quoted from Schenk, 2013, p. 1446). The manual control exercised by such senior officials can be preventive or reactive in emergency situations or conflicts and oriented toward top-down balancing of different interests, providing some benefits for followers and finding scapegoats if necessary. Usually, such analysis is concentrated on the federal system, but it also works at all levels when improvements depend on the personal decision of a top manager/administrator. In such a personified regime of regulation, informal institutions become more powerful and effective, based on multiple techniques, for example, the "telephone law" described by Alena Ledeneva. In the case of "telephone law," judicial independence is subverted for political purposes through "an informal command, request, or signal in order to influence formal procedures or decision-making" (Ledeneva, 2008, p. 326; Monaghan, 2012). In other words, a telephone call to the right person can result in a desired action by subverting official channels. Similarly, we conceptualize manual management as an informal instrument, applied by passing official (and often ineffective) rules.

We analyze personalized coordination in the Hospital (as well as in other hospitals) not so much as vertical way of overcoming formal rules but as horizontal connections to maintain formal rules on the operational level. Chiefs and heads of different departments and those in charge coordinate their decisions with each other when resources are insufficient, or the trajectory of a patient is unclear, or an unexpected inspection comes, etc. Therefore, we use the term "manual management" as referring not only to top-down control but also to the coordination and organization of routine work through maternity care providers' informal networks inside and outside the Hospital, which we recognize as one of their possible, and often-used, coping strategies.

There is also a similarity with manual control in the solution of both routine and emergency problems, which have to be solved personally, both in reactive and preventive ways. Maternity care providers opt for "telephone law" as well, though they try not to violate regular laws and rules, as control over them is rigid and severe. Solving numerous problems, they are not opposed to law, but try to find solutions in the "grey" zone of personal communication with colleagues, chiefs, and subordinators. Such management is implemented in order to accomplish contradictory notions of "good care," shaped by endless bureaucratic limitations and market demands. As previously noted, maternity care providers have to maintain the institutional order of the Hospital, make conditions workable and prevent patient complaints, maneuvering between different rules, orders and available resources. We will now show how these mechanisms work in different situations: when providers try to solve routine or critical problems of patients and when they prepare for expected inspections.

Manual management of routine problems

We often observed situations in the Hospital in which something was going wrong. For example, one woman came to the Hospital without appropriate papers. These are strictly demanded by official orders, but as she came from another city, her care providers there did not know about this and had not prepared these papers. She waited for hours in the emergency room while the head of the department tried to solve the problem by negotiating with those related to the problem, both within and outside the Hospital. Only top administrators could do this, because younger practitioners or administrators of lower level have no informal authority to negotiate such issues. The head said that those whom she should persuade are not easy to work with; the patient should receive a signature from another top administrator, who was going to a conference and agreed to communicate only after it was over. Finally, at the end of the day, we saw that the problem was solved as the woman received the permission, which the head had spent several hours to obtain.

During our research on whole working shifts in different departments, we observed how much coordination work had to be done by the departments' heads, their teams and other maternity care providers. One of our research participants was a head who solves numerous routine problems with regular treatment of patients and regulation of clinicians. In her words, she constructs logistical "chains" of different actors to achieve these goals, as formal rules are not sufficient to coordinate the complicated work of the Hospital, and thus systematic personal communication is needed, while her authority matters:

> *Working the shift with the chief. "Manual management". [During the day I observe that the] "chain" does combine different practitioners – that is permanent coordination of different cases, between physicians, and physicians and patients – construction of "chains". This work has little to do with formalized rules. Hierarchies are important, and it could not be done without the chief, who knows how and with whom to talk. I ask whether everything is coordinated like this, "yes" – she is smiling – "these are real chains". Women, physicians, nurses, midwives come to her clarify personally, call personally, ask personally.*
>
> *Not her secretary, but she herself should take care. She organizes special meetings, signs a lot of documents. Every moment somebody comes to her office or calls by phone to ask different questions: whether the pediatric service is interested in this case, when an obstetrician will return from maternity leave. Younger obstetricians have questions about records and other documents. She had about 40–50 incoming and outgoing calls per working day, mostly about coordination.*
>
> (field note)

We found some kind of node or checkpoint in every department, where the assemblage of different providers, patients, numerous documents, telephone calls and emotions are systematically enacted in coordination. The most visible is the registration office, but similar coordination work is ongoing in almost every department, and some routine problems are going to be solved there, often with the help of the head and the senior nurse:

> *[Our] shift in registration office. A lot of efforts are made to connect patients (especially with complicated problems) with physicians at wards, constant calls [from the office] to different departments and clinicians (obstetricians, pediatricians, neonatologist, cardiologists, anesthesiologists, etc.). Physicians, midwives, and heads often appear in the*

> *registration office to take care personally. . . . One record was lost, registrar promises the head will come and find the solution.*
>
> (field notes)

Another story was told by the head who tried to find extra beds for mothers of sick newborns. According to law, there should be the possibility for a mother to stay with her child, but there is no space and not enough beds in the Hospital. So, the head of department personally, and with the help of nurses, looked for additional beds and constantly negotiated with the different physicians and nurses in charge in order to get permission to locate mothers there. At the same time, she had to do emotional labor (see the next section) to console these women, as their children were in trouble.

While conducting ethnographic work, we observed manual management in many situations. For example, practitioners could agree with each other to buy some available medications by themselves for patients, as there is no legal possibility to do this quickly. In the laboratory, the technician said that providers often come themselves and wait for results to ensure that they are prioritized and done quickly. Manual management becomes especially evident in informal ways of personally coping with everyday problems derived from inconsistencies and bureaucratic obstacles that do not allow the provision of "good care":

> *They can cut [the expenses] or even delete [some items from the procurement list]. That's why my senior nurse is like a snake on a frying pan [in order to get what is needed for the department]. Borrows from these, takes this from that. Like in a big family.*
>
> (field notes, interview with Valentina, head of department)

Certainly, in every (not only Russian), context, maternity care providers communicate informally with each other, but in the context we studied, such communications did not aim only at solving clinical problems. Manual management is part and parcel of routine coordination within an inflexible healthcare system regulated by contradictory rules and multifaceted demands.

Manual management of critical problems

Maternity care providers in the Hospital had to implement a great deal of ad hoc coordination work in order to provide necessary medical care when they faced non-standard situations. In such Level 3 (high-ranking and technologically advanced) hospitals, there are many non-standard situations, as the most complicated cases from all the regions of the country are routed there. When faced with such complicated cases, providers have to activate all their resources and connections in order to help, but also must strive not to be sanctioned by the multiple controlling bodies. When we first asked why they could be punished, for example, for an unavoidable maternal death, they replied that there will be an obligatory investigation, which will always find something bureaucratically wrong, and someone has to be held responsible for this. We were surprised by this response, and asked "*Don't they [the State bodies who will investigate] know that you have to treat the most complicated cases?*" but no answer was given to this mostly rhetorical (for providers) question.

Obstetricians and pediatricians are often not supplied with resources and information (protocols or scripts) relevant to non-standard situations. For instance, we observed a woman who wanted to leave the Hospital before her treatment was over, due to a high level of mistrust to the physicians – she thought they were exaggerating the danger of her inborn heart condition. After the cesarean birth, she and her partner insisted on leaving the Hospital – despite the fact that she had been permanently in the ICU with this cardiovascular problem that endangered her life. We observed numerous negotiations between providers who cared about this woman, in which they discussed how to find a better approach and persuade her to behave "in a proper way." One physician assumed that the patient didn't realize the gravity of the threat, despite the fact that she was given endless medical explanations. Another obstetrician threatened to kick her husband out of the hospital. The chief and many practitioners firstly tried to persuade her not to leave the Hospital, but after very emotional and long-lasting negotiations with her and her partner, they decided to find a way to transfer her. The director made numerous calls to social service, the Ministry of Health, another hospital (where the chief personally knew the person in charge, but she was absent), and finally they managed to arrange to move her to another hospital, which was of a lower level, but was familiar to the patient. The woman agreed. The chief told us that if this woman died after leaving the Hospital, she (the chief) would be blamed anyway.

Manual management in coping with inspections

When inspection is expected, maternity care providers have to do a great deal of additional preparation in order to meet demands and to reduce the possible negative consequences. They explained to us that some rules could not be followed in a physical sense (some equipment, for example, does not fit in the physical space), and they had to negotiate with a colleague from another department in order to borrow equipment that does fit, for the limited time of inspection. The following example demonstrates a physical, logistical problem with the provision of meat to patients and the absence of a "proper" food cart. A nurse had to informally borrow a "proper" cart for the time of inspection, while everybody understood that this was impossible to do in a "proper" way:

> *Nurse in charge discusses with other nurses that there is no 'proper' food cart fitting normative standards, as such ["normative"] carts are inconvenient for transportations of food, and different ones are in use. "If you*

> *do according to the rules" – i.e. transport food in the correct containers and volumes – "there will be trash", because it is unrealistic to lift a heavy cart with full containers along the ramp – everything spills out.*
>
> (field notes)

> *But, as the inspector could check the right size and their temperature regime [according to normative standards], she tries to borrow the 'proper' food cart from another department, negotiating this with colleagues. She proposes to arrange a "demonstrative performance" with the proper cart (there is only one for the entire Hospital) so that it can be transported to all departments according to the rules, but this cart has no cover, and in this case, the temperature regime will be violated. "They'll kick ass anyway"; "Whatever the inspection, the sanction will follow."*
>
> (field notes)

Special work had to be done with patients before an inspector arrived. Here we provide an example of negotiation in the ward before the inspection, which is expected to control the "right order" in the Hospital. Nurses try to convince women to follow the rules of food storage, but patients do not want to follow those rules, which makes nurses add emotional tools – being disciplining, assertive and even rude (see the next section). The negotiations are emotional, and different actors – nurses and hospital's epidemiologists – expect complaints from women for their behavior, but the rules of food storage in the face of inspection are considered to be more important than women's needs:

> *We pass into the ward, nurse and the epidemiologist together scold the women in the ward (4 mothers), as they find food, including crackers. And such products are prohibited. Nurse to women: "Aren't you ashamed?" Epidemiologist: "If there is an infection, you will be transferred to another hospital!" Nurse: "I give time until 14.00. If there is no order, I will come with a garbage bag." Immediately throws away all the milk, cheese, and mayonnaise. The moms are clearly upset and are actively discussing the episode.*
>
> *(Outside the ward) Nurse 2: "I will not touch anything – mothers have already written a complaint against me that they are fed badly." Nurse 1: "Let them write a complaint about me" and loudly pronounces her name to the patients . . . Nurse 1 complains: "They write a complaint about the buffet too, this is the case in every ward! 'I would like to call the manager!' You are doing everything right, you have to teach, you have to throw it away."*
>
> (field notes)

As this example illustrates, working life in the Hospital consists of dozens of details that demand the personal involvement of providers in coordination – a manual management. We observed the exchanges of some equipment and drugs between departments – when they agreed with each other – running from one ward or department to another, or through negotiations with chiefs. In all such cases, providers had to initiate negotiations with colleagues and patients, and their success often depended on personal skills and personal relationships.

At the same time, childbearing women often do not notice or recognize this invisible work done by maternity care providers, and routinely find themselves in situations when their expectations are not met or something goes wrong for them, they do not understand the contradictory and volatile organizational rules (or the role of inspections) and explain their personal negative experiences in terms of professional failures, accusing obstetricians, pediatricians and nurses. Practitioners continually face and permanently expect grievances from patients, and have to manage emerging problems manually in order to navigate a woman within the complicated organizational system of the Hospital and help her to get all the assistance and services that she needs, or in order to fit institutional order and rules. Conditions and rules of health organizations often do not meet assertive patients' demands, nor do the requirements of controlling bodies, and providers have to meet these multiple challenges within the inflexible institutional setting. They rarely have enough autonomy to negotiate treatment with women; they have no resources, formal protocols or scripts to overcome contradictory bureaucratic rules and withstand women' growing demands. So, they solve problems through personified coordination – manual management, telephone law – and various communicative practices.

In the quite complicated process of manual management, the need to work as a team takes on a special meaning. Members in personalized relationships should trust each other; otherwise this system of negotiations fails. Practitioner's personality matters, and belonging to the trusting circle (being "*svoi*," see Chapter 2) becomes a very important category within the Hospital in particular and the system of maternity care in general. But the downside is that if there is a conflict or lack of trust among participants, the system malfunctions. In such conditions, childbearing women are considered as "obstacles" if they do not obey and follow instructions, both clinical and logistical. Maternity care providers express nostalgic feelings about the previous respect they received from (normatively) obedient childbearing women during the Soviet era. Obstetricians under market pressure have to meet patients' demands and provide "good care," while dealing with new professional tasks and standards. Under these multiple pressures, providers have had to renegotiate their new roles, including the increasingly articulated necessity to provide emotional support to women. This invisible "grey zone" constitutes the space for clinicians' autonomy, within which they try to provide as much "good care" as they can. But in such conditions, they themselves become vulnerable subjects.

Maternity care providers' emotional labor

Emotional labor in the Hospital is framed by more general emotional styles, which are now changing and being reflexively negotiated in Russian healthcare. We understand "emotional style" (Illouz, 2007) here as the configuration of prescribed emotional rules and emotions performed on the level of professional-patient interactions, shaped by organizational and institutional contexts and entangled with multiple modes of care. The previously taken-for-granted Soviet rudeness (*khamstvo*) and disregard in maternity care are now challenged by new professional standards and consumers' demands for supportive care (see Temkina et al., 2021). A new style of *smiling* emerges. To dig deeper into this process, we will explore which techniques providers use to deal with the emotions of others and how they juggle among these various techniques.

We conceptualize the emotional practices of *khamstvo* and *smiling* as the dominant, contrasting, signifiers (the most notable parts of the repertoires) of Soviet and post-Soviet emotional styles in maternity care. *Khamstvo* was taken for granted in Soviet maternity care as a way of performing obstetricians' situational power over childbearing women. We agree with Rivkin-Fish (2005) that *khamstvo* used to be an important tool to discipline and control women, place them under clinicians' authority and shape the attitudes of all participants, including the maternity care practitioners themselves, who often claimed to feel helpless in the rigid State paternalistic hierarchies. "Ignorant" and "infantile" (according to obstetricians' definitions) women are forced to cooperate and behave in the right way during delivery "for the sake of the mother's and child's health." We observed situations in which obstetricians raised their voices and expressed threats when care receivers refused to follow instructions or insisted on their own opinion.

Maternity care providers are confident in their rights to subordinate women to their will, as the Russian system of maternity care demands this from them. Obstetricians justified their behavior as an effort to prevent patients from acting in a way considered wrong or shameful during the medical encounter, and therefore did not see it as *khamstvo*. (In Chapter 4, we explored how women tried to avoid such a rude style of communication.) The new, emotionally sensitive style of politeness (smiling) has emerged due to the development of neoliberal consumer capitalism in Russia, and in maternity care in particular. The ongoing shift in Russian institutional settings can be characterized as changing toward "the display and embrace of 'positive' emotions . . . while it requires the control and management of 'negative' ones" (Sieben & Wettergren, 2010, p. 4). This new kind of emotional labor is also forced by the need to mitigate women's inconveniences caused by systematic institutional uncertainties. Providers state that they should manage their emotions in order to avoid conflicts; they do a lot of emotional labor in order to mitigate women's grievances that might otherwise lead to emotional outbursts and consequent complaints. Obstetricians, neonatologists, nurses and midwives implement specific strategies that allow for the preventive management of complaints or prevent their escalation. We will show that two styles as two modes of care (rudeness and politeness) co-exist in healthcare institutions and that social actors are juggling between them.

Emotional labor as a coping strategy for inconsistencies: juggling different techniques

The changes that took place after the Soviet collapse have shaped the rules and repertoires of emotional practices in hospitals. Nowadays, providers use the tools of different emotional styles. While *smiling* became a required, consumer-oriented emotional work to be accomplished, *khamstvo* is still reported as a familiar emotional practice. Obstetricians and midwives explain the reason for *khamstvo* as resulting from the "inappropriate" reactions of women. They say that some patients become extra demanding and aggressive; they are noncompliant, service-oriented and expecting unrealistic service, infantile and care-requiring.

Obstetricians sometimes feel that it is appropriate to raise their voices and act rudely and forcefully (*khamstvo*) not only because they cannot fully do the emotional labor and control their reactions but also because they see that as the only way to make women obey their rules and prescriptions. In case the women don't, the negative medical consequences will be qualified as the obstetrician's fault (with all the legal consequences): "*What can I do, how can I not raise my voice and not shout if she does not listen and does not obey me?*" (field note, conversation with an obstetrician). In such situations when obstetricians try to persuade women, they perceive a degree of *khamstvo* as a legitimate technique. The emotional style of *khamstvo* is structurally reproduced through attitudes of paternalism and an asymmetrical balance of power. Importantly, in these situations, providers rarely consider these kinds of behavior as *khamstvo*.

Providers assume that in taking legal and professional responsibility and acting for the sake of clients, they can legitimately neglect women's emotional needs and subordinate them to clinical and organizational conditions through direct rude orders and "negative" emotional work. As previously noted, obstetricians sometimes use aggressive techniques to persuade patients, in order to minimize medical and administrative risks and to subordinate patients to their decisions. They say that they also have to implement the role of disciplining agent when women are "ignorant" and "irresponsible," do not want to follow instructions, quarrel with doctors and midwives and have "no relevant knowledge." Such women, according to maternity care providers, are not prepared for childbirth, do not want to take responsibility and articulate "irrelevant" demands. One obstetrician said, "*They want us do all their labor in delivery*" (field notes). According to providers, the growth in patients' access to information does not indicate competence or good preparation for childbirth.

Obstetricians are convinced that, as experts, they are the only ones with reliable knowledge; they see themselves as knowledgeable and responsible, but also as those who have to make special efforts to control women's behavior, to correct and teach the ignorant, "childlike" patients how to behave properly. In such cases, obstetricians consider themselves as implementing paternalistic quasi-parenting. They typically reaffirm medical paternalism as a foundational part of expert authority and "good care," which ultimately legitimates their power over childbearing women.

We observed other situations in which obstetricians raised their voices and expressed threats when patients refused to follow instructions or insisted on their own opinion:

> *Physicians exert pressure (on the woman). They raise their voices. Then the doctor tells me: "They [the woman and her husband] will go to complain. We can expect nasty things, she will write to the President."*
> (field notes)

In Soviet maternity care, women blamed providers for *khamstvo*, yet nowadays both care receivers and providers can accuse each other of *khamstvo* and feel a legitimate "right" to discipline the other side, as the distribution of power in their interactions is quite complicated. Rude emotional work is performed by medical practitioners toward women, and vice versa:

> *He [the women's husband] wrote such a devastating complaint against a physician, kind of "what a khamka (boor)!"... She [the physician] already had such complaints, in general... She is a good specialist, but she is well... sometimes very... well, a little bit bitchy.*
> (interview with Varvara Alekseevna, head of department)

In this case, the head of the department accuses another practitioner of *khamstvo*, which appears to be a category that can be subjectively attributed to any participant in the communication. We see how being "a good specialist" and using rude communication techniques can co-exist. While *khamstvo* is perceived very negatively by patients, using it does not put into question the professional competencies of physicians

However, maternity care practitioners have to provide positive emotional labor as well. Mothers-to-be in their new consumer roles have become assertive and expect more "positive" emotional work to be done in maternity care. Providers are required to display service-style smiling, which presupposes the consumer orientation of childbearing women, whose needs should be taken into account. Again, providers have to manage their emotions to avoid patient complaints, emotional outbursts, and conflicts. Control over emotions has become a regulated part of professional display in maternity hospitals. As providers put it, it is necessary to "*control your emotions*" (field notes, conversation with nurse), and problematic situations "*need to be smoothed somehow*" (interview with Anastasia, midwife). Maternity care practitioners now learn communicative and emotional skills. An obstetrician confirms: *But there is no other way out: if you don't talk [to a patient], she will go to the chief ones. She will go to complain* (interview with Mila, head of department).

In a specific communicational situation, different practices can accompany each other, so that the same situation can appear to be split. Here is one example of an interaction we observed at our field site:

> *The woman in labor screams while the obstetrician (ob) manually opens the cervix [an excruciatingly painful and usually unnecessary procedure]. The obstetrician speaks in a raised voice.*
>
> *Ob: [Ira], what are you doing? You are an adult.*
> *Ira: It hurts!*
> *Ob: It's not that painful.*
> *Ira: Please, don't press like that!*
> *Ob: I am not pressing. You are the one trying to find a way out.*
> *Ira: I can't!*
> *Ob: You can, you can. Now the anesthesiologists will come and they will save you [give epidural analgesia]. If you do not obey me, then none of this will work. You don't have to resist.*
> *Ira: I understand. But I cannot.*
> *Ob: "I can't" are the wrong words. You must say "I can."*
>
> (field notes)

In this case, the obstetrician was constantly balancing between different emotional styles. Sometimes she used denominations that displayed care in order to make the woman cooperate ("kitten," "you can do that," "you are my princess," "a smart girl"). In other situations, like the one described in the previous field note, she required obedience instead of cooperation, didn't explain the details of the procedure and tried to downplay the patient's suffering ("not that painful"). Her disregard for the patient's experience is further evidenced by the likelihood that she could have explained why she couldn't manually dilate the cervix after the epidural was administered (there were certain clinical reasons for that). This is not pure *khamstvo*, but a hybrid of both *khamstvo* and *smiling*, paternalism ("doctor knows best"), and consumerism (women can choose – e.g., for pain relief, a laboring woman can use the birthing ball, take a long shower, or get an epidural, and have a partner next to her). In a private discussion later on, the obstetrician explained that this patient required special attention due to some medical complications, and also assured us how much she loves her job. In this sense, maternity care providers have become "emotional jugglers," moving between women's consumer demands, requirements imposed by administration and State officials, and institutional limitations.

Maternity care providers' emotions and vulnerabilities

Providers perform multifaceted "good care" by widening their professional roles and implementing various techniques of coping with inconsistencies; these are time-consuming and difficult tasks. The requirements, dictated by notions of "good care" on different levels, are difficult to satisfy, which leads to the growth of complaints from patients and increasing sanctions from controlling State bodies. Thus, providers feel themselves vulnerable when coping with multiple challenges: complicated clinical tasks, being controlled by different State bodies, and the emotional responses of patients. Our data show that maternity care providers can feel vulnerable when they encounter "unfair" (in their terms) interpretations and evaluations of their actions, and they expect sanctions and accusations. Vulnerability arises when practitioners are assigned responsibility for situations they cannot control, and when they get "baseless" complaints from patients. Unfair claims from patients and from regulatory bodies can have legal consequences that create both symbolic and real threats. Practitioners are also aware of their helplessness when faced with the inability to save or cure a patient or her baby.

Despite the fact that biomedicine objectively cannot save everyone, practitioners tend to take negative outcomes (deaths or severe birth complications) personally. This is exacerbated by the fact that in reproductive medicine, death or the threat of death can occur to "nonconventional" demographic groups (the ones who "should not" die) – young women and newborns. Practitioners explained to us that they will keep on trying to save a patient even in a hopeless clinical situation, or in situations with negative prognoses. In cases of lethal outcomes, they feel their helplessness, and this experience leaves lifelong scars:

> *At the intern's room, we find out who passed away in the last week. A woman, right after the operation, a severe pathology, delivery at 34th week (pregnancy was contraindicated), the newborn has probably survived. There are no [official] complaints yet.*
>
> (field notes)

Despite the fact that this situation was predictable (this became clear later, during the clinical examination of the case) and wasn't followed up by relatives' complaints or a lawsuit, many physicians got engaged, and the case was widely discussed as stressful for them. This woman's physical condition carried fatal risks – "*It was inevitable, there were no medical mistakes*" (field notes, conversation with head of department).

Different departments deal with challenging cases, deaths and the emotions of patients to different extents. For instance, the emergency room or consultative-diagnostic department would dramatically differ from maternity ward or intensive care units (ICUs):

> *Obstetricians always fight at the forefront for life and death.*
>
> (field notes, conversation with neonatologist)

> *If for other departments clinical death is a stress, for us it's a job. We are the most stressed department.*
>
> (field notes, conversation with ICU nurse)

Maternity care providers in the Hospital specialize in working with severe clinical cases; therefore mortality, bad outcomes and poor clinical prognoses are inevitable parts of their work. However, maternity care providers speak about severe cases or loss with personal emotional involvement. They are worried and frustrated, and it is hard for them to tolerate every case of maternal or neonatal death. Such situations are sensitive for those who are involved, not only because they can be legally prosecuted in cases of death of a patient or serious harm to her – which they could do nothing about – but also because they often do not have enough authority and trust in the eyes of patients to protect them from making wrong decisions about their health, and maternity care practitioners must take personal responsibility for this.

Along with the emotional challenges that their profession brings, maternity care providers constantly feel themselves as objects of all-around control. They speak about their precarity and insecurity under the State's "controlling gaze," which is perceived as a threat to their professional status and personhood in general. Threat is a kind of "outer force" ("*God forbid something happens*," a neonatologist said), which lies beyond the professional's control and creates feelings of hopelessness and helplessness. Obstetricians metaphorically refer to George Orwell (1949): "*Big brother is watching you*" (field notes), meaning overall control. During our fieldwork, we regularly observed maternity care practitioners discussing future inspections and the dangers they can bring:

> *I say – [this is] a personal insecurity . . . nobody will be on our side, nobody will help.*
>
> (interview with Varvara Alekseevna, head of department)

> *Nobody will protect physicians . . . nobody advocates for physicians in front of the public.*
>
> (field notes)

The feeling that everyone could be accused of something makes maternity care providers feel defenseless in front of controlling bodies. The provision of "good care" forces them to negotiate around formal rules and recommendations, and sometimes to break them. Consequently, they can potentially be accused or sanctioned. Physicians clearly understand this, and say with a sad irony that: "*My task is to prepare everything for the prosecutor, so that he can't get to me*" (field notes, interview with Valentina, head of department).

As previously noted, the contemporary demographic pronatalist politics of the State are directed toward increasing the birth rate and thus attract a great deal of State attention to maternity care. As a result, every case of maternal mortality (regardless of its inevitability) has become an issue for special attention from controlling and law-enforcement bodies and a potential legal threat to all maternity care providers who were involved in the process of treatment. Such control is becoming more pervasive due to the new instruments, such as audio and video recordings of sessions with providers made by patients, the creation of online sites for evaluation of providers' and medical organizations' performance and the elaboration of legal channels for dealing with patients' requests and complaints about the quality of medical care. Patients are complaining more, and maternity care providers are taking this hard, as it can lead to additional inspections, administrative and material sanctions, reputational losses and emotional costs. The obstetrician who was mentioned in the complaint was taking the situation very hard and was even about to quit her job:

> *There were two proceedings [after the complaint]. The obstetrician had been going crazy all five days before that. She was sending messages to me: "Maybe I should quit my job?" . . . Reputationally this is very painful.*
>
> (interview with Elena Vladimirovna, director of the Hospital)

Practitioners are bothered because every patient can record a conversation and post it on the internet: "*Patients are taking pictures of us with their mobile phones, and we feel and consider this*" (field notes, conversation with a nurse).

For an obstetrician who is herself struggling with a threatening sanction, it is difficult to provide sufficient support to suffering patients or their relatives. As a result of the lack of mutual trust, practitioners are urged to use affective and "forceful" arguments, while patients respond to these with aggression and even greater mistrust. In the aforementioned situation in which a woman insisted on leaving the Hospital despite her obstetrician's and cardiologist's strong recommendations to the contrary, she mistrusted the given recommendations. A wide spectrum of medical care providers, who felt themselves responsible both for her life and for the good of her newborn, were experiencing a mix of strong emotions, from anger to desperation. As Anna Temkina observed:

> *[Physicians] are speaking quite roughly . . . It was emotionally hard for me, maybe because of the hopelessness of the situation and inability to negotiate . . . Verbally physicians are threatening and bullying her to make her stay (and continue treatment). Although – no doubt – they make it for her benefit and maybe even saving her life. [One of them] doesn't sleep at night.*
>
> (field notes)

Maternity care practitioners have to provide emotional labor on a daily basis, to cope with their own strong emotions derived from the vulnerability of their positions and to satisfy women's expectations of warm, personalized care and an emotionally satisfying childbirth experience. Such practitioners feel themselves vulnerable due to their structural positions and high levels of responsibility. They are expected to perform multiple tasks that they were not prepared for – as we have seen, they have to walk in the shoes of managers, psychologists, bureaucrats, etc. There are many organizational inconsistencies and controversies between different ideals of "good care," but providers still can be accused of performing them wrongly or badly. They are constantly frustrated by the facts that they can be legally accused, that they will dissatisfy consumerist expectations, or will be ineffective. At the same time, their own professional duties presuppose many emotional challenges; they literally face issues of life and death, with which they have to cope. All those together make maternity care providers feel themselves vulnerable and their own profession as precarious and non-prestigious.

Conclusion: between a rock and a hard place

Maternity care providers in Russia are bouncing between the State and market demands. New professional tasks emerge in this hybrid system: along with maternity care provision, practitioners have to cope with strict bureaucratic rules (managerial logic), new high professional standards of care (professional logic) and growing patients' consumeristic demands (market logic). Multiple pressures affect their structural positions – making them less autonomous and more vulnerable – and their working practices, requiring meeting multifaceted expectations and demands.

"Good care" in maternity services becomes a subject of constant negotiations within and between different actors. The State bodies, professional groups, and patients participate in (re)defining "good care." Perspectives vary greatly, as they refer to different logics, ideas and practices. Maternity care providers have to deal with all of them and, hence, simultaneously be concerned with governmental demographic politics; show efficiency and reduce the expenses of treatment; strictly obey the rigid rules; and be attentive to the personal needs of patients and their families. To do all of this at once is logistically and practically impossible – they are trapped "between a rock and a hard place" – yet they feel they must try. As a result, they have to maneuver between different professional roles, communicative and emotional practices, and coping strategies in medical encounters.

In the context of the Soviet legacy, which includes paternalism toward patients and their families, it could be supposed that Russian maternity care providers are used to powerful positions. However, we argue just the opposite: that State paternalism enhances the vulnerabilities of Russian healthcare providers with lack of authority, of professional autonomy and of the resources needed to provide "good care." The autonomy and ability to make clinical decisions for obstetricians are challenged by the demands formed by market and State. At the same time, the scope of their professional roles and obligations expands; they are expected to provide psychological, emotional and administrative support to their patients.

Again, the requirements, dictated by multifaceted notions of "good care" on different levels, are logistically and practically impossible to satisfy, and this systematically leads to the growth of complaints from patients and sanctions from controlling State bodies. Maternity care practitioners feel themselves vulnerable and routinely cope with multiple challenges by manual management – in order to provide "good care," they have to constantly negotiate, do extra work and customize themselves to situations that lie beyond the clinical agenda. They are trying to satisfy the requirements and expectations by using personalized navigation of patients in an entangled, bureaucratized system; horizontal informal communication and exchange within and between departments; constantly adapting current settings to maladaptive, rigid and top-down regulatory rules. They have to juggle between different emotional practices in order to prevent complaints and meet new consumer demands for personalized care, at the same time as they still feel that they must subordinate women to clinical and organizational conditions – primarily to protect themselves from official negative sanctions, but at the same time opening themselves up to consumer complaints – yet another trap between a rock and a hard place.

The new emotional neoliberal style of *smiling* does not radically change the balance of power, the structural norms or the contradictory rules that beleaguer medical organizations, though it does work to humanize their applications. The rude style of *khamstvo* is still there. Maternity care providers typically reaffirm medical paternalism as a foundational part of expert authority that ultimately legitimates their power over childbearing women. The emotional practices associated with *khamstvo* are employed in such situations, even though they no longer comprise the dominant style of communication and are not fully accepted as routine anymore. Nowadays, different and contradicting emotional styles coexist in Russian maternity care, and the participants – obstetricians, neonatologists, midwives, nurses, administrators and all those who work in the field of maternity care, along with women and their partners – must navigate in the complex emotional and bureaucratic landscape that constitutes maternity care in contemporary Russia.

In sum, the coping strategies of Russian maternity care providers include manual management and emotional labor, as they have to balance between formal rules, State requirements and care receivers' expectations. In so doing, they generate multiple informal techniques but cannot significantly change the rules and norms of the entire field of maternity care. However, in some cases, they aim at changing the institutional arrangement of maternity services. The following chapter addresses this issue, analyzing how professional projects can become strategic political actions.

Note

1 Doulas are non-medical specialists who provide emotional support and caring practices for women during pregnancy, birth and the postpartum period.

References

Borozdina, E. (2014). The social organization of natural childbirth: The case of center for midwifery care. *Journal of Social Policy Studies*, 12(3), 413–426.

Borozdina, E. (2016). Zabota v rodovspomozhenii: vygody i izderzhki professionalov [Professional care in maternity hospitals: Benefits and challenges]. *Zhurnal Issledovaniy Sotsial'noy Politiki [The Journal of Social Policy Studies]*, 14(4), 479–492.

Borozdina, E., & Novkunskaya, A. (2020). Patient-centered care in Russian maternity hospitals: Introducing a new approach through professionals' agency. *Health: An Interdisciplinary Journal for the Social Study of Health, Illness and Medicine*, 1–21. https://doi.org/10.1177/1363459320925871.

Davis-Floyd, R. (2001). The technocratic, humanistic, and holistic paradigms of childbirth. *International Journal of Gynecology & Obstetrics*, 75(S5).

Davis-Floyd, R. (2018). The technocratic, humanistic, and holistic paradigms of birth and health care. In R. Davis-Floyd & L. Grove (Eds.), *Ways of Knowing about Birth: Mothers, Midwives, Medicine, and Birth Activism* (pp. 3–44). Long Grove, IL: Waveland Press.

Davis-Floyd, R. E., & Cheyney, M. (2022). *Birth as an American Rite of Passage* (3rd ed.). Abingdon, Oxon: Routledge.

Fotaki, M. (2013). Is patient choice the future of health care systems? *International Journal of Health Policy and Management*, 1(2), 121–123.

Fotaki, M. (2014). Can consumer choice replace trust in the National Health Service in England? Towards developing an affective psychosocial conception of trust in health care. *Sociology of Health & Illness*, 36(8), 1276–1294.

Freidson, E. (1970). *Profession of Medicine; A Study of the Sociology of Applied Knowledge*. New York: Dodd, Mead.

Freidson, E. (2001). *Professionalism, the Third Logic: On the Practice of Knowledge*. Chicago: University of Chicago Press.
Gabe, J., Harley, K., & Calnan, M. (2015). Healthcare choice: Discourses, perceptions, experiences and practices. *Current Sociology*, 63(5), 623–635.
Hochschild, A. R. (1983). *The Managed Heart: Commercialization of Human Feeling*. Berkeley: University of California Press.
Illouz, E. (2007). *Cold Intimacies*. Cambridge: Polity Press.
Ledeneva, A. (2008). Telephone justice in Russia. *Post-Soviet Affairs*, 24(4), 324–350.
Lipsky, M. (1980). *Street-level Bureaucracy: Dilemmas of the Individual in Public Services*. New York: Russell Sage Foundation.
Litvina, D., Novkunskaya, A., & Temkina, A. (2020). Multiple vulnerabilities in medical settings: Invisible suffering of doctors. *Societies*, 10(1), 5.
Lupton, D. (1997). Consumerism, reflexivity and the medical encounter. *Social Science & Medicine*, 45(3), 373–381.
Ministry of Health of the Russian Federation. (2020). *The Order "On Approval of the Procedure for Providing Medical Care in the Profile" Obstetrics and Gynecology*. N 1130n of 20.10.2020. Available at: https://base.garant.ru/74840123/ (Accessed 19.07.22).
Monaghan, A. (2012). The vertikal: Power and authority in Russia. *International Affairs*, 88(1), 1–16.
Orwell, G. (1949). *Ninteen Eighty-four: A Novel*. New York: Harcourt, Brace and Company.
Ozhiganova, A. A. (2020). 'Aktivnoye nedoveriye' vracham: sluchay yuridicheskogo soprovozhdeniya rodov ['Active mistrust' of doctors: A case of legal support in childbirth]. *Sibirskiye istoricheskiye issledovaniya [Siberian Historical Research]*, 4, 195–215 (In Russian).
Ozhiganova, A. A., & Molodtsova, M. O. (2020). Rody v usloviyakh karantina: pozitsiya douly [Quarantined childbirth: Doula's position]. *Meditsinskaya antropologiya i bioetika [Medical Anthropology and Bioethics]*, 1(19), 158–173.
Parsons, T. (2013 [1951]). *The Social System*. London: Routledge.
Petrov, N., Lipman, M., & Hale, H. E. (2010). Overmanaged democracy in Russia: Governance implications of hybrid regimes. *Carnegie Papers*. Washington, DC: Carnegie Endowment for International Peace.
Petrov, N., Lipman, M., & Hale, H. E. (2014). Three dilemmas of hybrid regime governance: Russia from Putin to Putin. *Post-Soviet Affairs*, 30(1), 1–26. http://doi.org/10.1080/1060586X.2013.825140.
Rivkin-Fish, M. R. (2005). *Women's Health in Post-Soviet Russia: The Politics of Intervention*. Bloomington: Indiana University Press.
Saks, M. (2015). *The Professions, State and the Market: Medicine in Britain, the United States and Russia*. Abingdon, New York: Routledge.
Schenk, C. (2013). Controlling immigration manually: Lessons from Moscow (Russia). *Europe-Asia Studies*, 65(7), 1444–1465.
Scott, W. R., Ruef, M., Mendel, P. J., & Caronna, C. A. (2000). *Institutional Change and Healthcare Organizations: From Professional Dominance to Managed Care*. Chicago: University of Chicago Press.
Sieben, B., & Wettergren, Å. (2010). Emotionalizing organizations and organizing emotions – our research agenda. In B. Sieben & Å. Wettergren (Eds.),

Emotionalizing Organizations and Organizing Emotions (pp. 1–20). London: Palgrave MacMillan.

Temkina, A. (2019). 'Childbirth is not a car rental': Mothers and obstetricians negotiating consumer service in Russian commercial maternity care. *Critical Public Health*, 30(5), 521–532.

Temkina, A., Litvina, D., & Novkunskaya, A. (2021). Emotional styles in Russian maternity hospitals: Juggling between khamstvo and smiling. *Emotions and Society*, 3(1), 95–113.

Tummers, L. L., Bekkers, V., Vink, E., & Musheno, M. (2015). Coping during public service delivery: A conceptualization and systematic review of the literature. *Journal of Public Administration Research and Theory*, 25(4), 1099–1126.

Chapter 6

Struggling for "good care"

The professional as political

Nowadays in Russia, new initiatives are emerging in maternity care that advocate for the improvement of care and the empowerment of both practitioners and childbearing women. While practitioners' influences on maternity care (and more broadly on healthcare) seem to be very local, we argue that eventually these social actors challenge and change the field of maternity care by incrementally introducing their own principles of "good care."

In this chapter, we present empirical findings from several cases related to rank-and-file initiatives of maternity care providers: professional associations, trade unions and non-governmental organizations (NGO). We ask and answer the questions of what kinds of initiatives can be undertaken under strict administrative control, limited professional autonomy, market pressures, and the absence of an influential women's and consumers' movement: who are the key actors of such initiatives, and what are their strategies and results? We argue that these key actors advocate for changes in maternity care provision and challenge the current state of affairs ("*the System*"). We use the idea that "the professional is political" in ways similar to the feminist "the personal is political" agenda that has been articulated by women's movements since the 1970s. We employ both feminist and "strategic action field" approaches in order to conceptually frame our arguments.

In this chapter, we first refer to the ongoing struggles of Russian midwives for professional autonomy and status through independent initiatives, associations, professional initiatives and debates, based on our own data and the research of our colleagues. We then proceed to a case analysis of the rebellion of maternity care practitioners against changes in their working conditions in a small town; this rebellion generated an alliance with an independent trade union of medical practitioners. And then we turn to non-governmental philanthropy related to the perinatal sphere, particularly to perinatal palliative care and reproductive losses. In conclusion, we summarize how such initiatives turn *professional* issues in Russia into *political* ones.

DOI: 10.4324/9781003139539-6

Professionals' political and strategic actions

As we have shown in previous chapters, most of the large-scale transformations in Russian healthcare have occurred in a top-down mode, and providers have had to adapt to these changes. This vertical bureaucratic control in Russia presupposes political loyalty as the basis of sustainability, access to resources and institutional safety. Therefore, demonstrations of loyalty and acceptance of current rules appear to be important institutional norms, which are followed by "*incumbents.*" As we showed in Chapter 5, social actors in maternity care are constantly maneuvering among different demands and coordinating routine activities through manual management, and sometimes change conditions by default, without the bottom-up *public voicing* that we address in this chapter. Yet voice from below is possible as professionals become aware of numerous health and maternity care problems and of problems in their positioning. Some of them find possibilities for improvement and empower themselves as actors capable of changes. Maternity care providers recognize their professional problems as both political and systemic (all of them refer to "the System"), or structurally determined; thus, we define the process of changing the established order as "political" in a broad sense.

Other scholars also define the professional as political – for instance, to explore how social workers empower their clients (Hartman, 1993); how counselors participate in system-level change on behalf of clients (Arthur & Collin, 2014); or how micropolitics in professional knowledge and practice are implemented in psychotherapy (Rossiter, 2000). Davis-Floyd and Johnson (2006) refer to "the professional as political" regarding midwives in the United States, who must deeply engage in politics as they struggle in various states for legislation and regulations that empower them and do not restrict their practices. The feminist agenda is referred to in institutional critiques of academia as excluding the voices of women of color (Edmonds, 2019). Also, the labor and knowledge of professionals working in such fields as science, education or law come from certain standpoints and entail ideas on the "collective good" and ways to achieve it. Therefore, their professional activities on different levels are framed as political. The saying, "the professional is political" is applied broadly at the levels of institutional and professional micro-politics and refers to topics related to power (im)balance, inequality and societal changes. This perspective is critically opposed to the supposedly *apolitical* neutrality of expert knowledge and professional institutions.

Medical professions are also involved in struggles for power and are not neutral. For example, Inna Leykin and Michele Rivkin-Fish (2022) demonstrate these elements in their research on obstetricians' engagements with politicized demography and pronatalist politics in Russia (see also Nakachi, 2021). Not only are *"challengers"* of the System political actors but also conservative professionals (as we denote here – *incumbents*) may influence or be influenced by politics. Obstetricians worldwide are involved in abortion policy-making; in Soviet society they have popularized an anti-abortion agenda. In this way, they (*professionally*) advocate for preserving women's health and (*politically*) follow the State agenda. In Russia, physicians react to national demographic goals and intentionally promote ideas about women's emotional health and wellbeing as relevant to the State priorities of pronatalist demographic goals: healthy women will give birth to healthy children.

Thus, professional power on the structural level can be maintained, along with State politics and loyalty to the System, though this does not lead directly to power for the rank-and-file maternity care providers. Professional power can also be achieved through the promotion of changes from below in maternity care; we are especially interested in this particular political dimension as the space for positive change and empowerment of providers and, consequently, their clients. What makes changes from below into agentive political acts is that they are being realized in the contexts of bureaucratic paternalist State power, limited space for professional autonomy, and restrictions on vocalizing oppositional political opinions. Herein we will be looking at the strategic actions on the meso level that are taken by some groups and organizations in the field of maternity care. In order to conceptualize new initiatives of maternity care professionals as political (oriented toward changes) and as empowering practitioners to improve care, we refer to the conceptual model of the "strategic action field" (SAF) (Fligstein & McAdam, 2011). We use this framework in order to understand how the struggle for "good care" from below could lead to changes in maternity care, which is rigidly regulated by the State, on the one side, and inhabited by multiple and competing social actors on the other. We note that the main sites of changes are the legal institutions of maternity care (maternity hospitals, first of all), though different actors can be involved in transformations, and we also use some tools of organizational theory in order to elaborate our arguments about processes in the "organizational field."

In terms of organizational theory and the sociology of social movements, we conceptualize maternity care in Russia as an *organizational field* embracing the network of relations among different collective and individual actors: nurses, midwives, physicians, administrators, professional associations, researchers, students, informal groups, allies, new attendants, women, etc. A variety of actors interact in any organizational field: "Individuals, groups, divisions of an organization, firms, universities, nonprofits, social movement organizations, departments or ministries in governments, states, and intergovernmental organizations" (Fligstein, 2008, pp. 6–7). Together, such actors constitute a non-coherent but stable order that includes unequal distribution of power and resources.

The possibilities for actors to have control differ, and such actors are also differently positioned in relation to institutional stability or change. Some actors (incumbents) are working on guarding that stability and preserving existing power relations, while others (challengers) act to relocate resources in a given context and to undertake strategic actions to possess more control over the core of the field (Fligstein & McAdam, 2011, p. 5). In this chapter, challengers will be our focus; we analyze their strategic actions as political – aimed at "changing the rules of the game," or at social changes in the field of maternity care. Challengers do not unreflexively follow shared institutional rules but challenge them and work to change the organizational settings in which they work.

The possibilities for change are limited by both internal and external factors. Social, economic and cultural contexts exert influence on arrangements and interactions, as well as on the allocation of resources. Possibilities for change differ between the center and the periphery. As we explained in Chapter 3, the State plays the crucial central role in controlling the rules and compliance with them, while other key actors possess major control in the field of maternity care, acting either to support the existing order or its top-down reformation. The possibilities for challengers to generate change are limited and often innovative; that is why we are especially interested in their successful (or not) strategies, elaborated in order to change the rules of the existing organizational order in maternity care, or the order itself. Their strategies differ; their repertoire includes semi-legal practices outside and inside official facilities, grassroots efforts within maternity hospitals, activities in professional associations, the public voicing of protests and NGO activities promoting "good care."

The challengers in the field of maternity care elaborate alternative approaches and rules to regulate relations between maternity care receivers and care providers; they challenge the existing order. Here we focus on those groups of challengers who take not only strategic but also "innovative actions, which have not been used widely before" (Fligstein & McAdam, 2011, p. 9). This is the "field of struggle," as the majority of institutional incumbents prefer to sustain the existing institutional order and its rules.

To make different cases of these innovative actors inhabiting the field of maternity care provision relatively comparable, our description of each case will proceed according to the following questions:

- Actors: Who (individually or collectively) in a group or organization acts as challenger(s) of the existing rules regulating maternity care provision?
- Strategies: What actions are actually taken to challenge the status quo of the field? What kinds of resources are employed to realize the strategy? How does mobilization happen, and what alliances and networks are established to achieve change?
- Relation to the State: How do these actors relate to the "governance units," both within and outside the maternity care field?
- Symbolic dimensions of initiatives: What kinds of cognitive constructs and collectively shared meanings (*conceptions of control*) emerge in

the field via the actions of the challengers? How do ideas about "good care" emerge and motivate their struggles?

- Results: How have the challengers' actions changed the field of maternity care?

Midwives and doulas struggling for "good care": semi-formal initiatives entering hospitals

As previously noted, neither midwives nor nurses have professional autonomy or independent practice in post-Soviet Russian institutionalized maternity care (and in healthcare more generally). Legally, they can only assist obstetricians or other physicians, following their instructions. The idea of "professional autonomy" appeared in Russia in the late 1990s in some special niches of independent, alternative, spiritual and homebirth practices of midwives and doulas who were prone to introduce and elaborate innovative approaches, but at the same time used to have and still have limited access to official maternity care institutions (Borozdina, 2014a, b, 2017, 2018; Ozhiganova, 2019a, b).

In the USSR, the homebirth movement emerged in the 1980s, and has developed significantly since the 1990s (Beloussova, 2002; Ozhiganova, 2019a, c), as new requests appeared from childbearing women who were not satisfied with the maternity services provided in State-funded facility-based settings (see Chapter 3). This movement was not coherent, obtained no legal status, and its radical projects of maternity care's transformation appeared unsustainable; sometimes homebirth midwives were legally prosecuted. In addition, these initiatives developed mostly in small midwifery projects, sometimes called centers, where women legally could only be prepared for hospital birth (and not give birth, at least officially), or emerged in forms of independent consultations in different areas. These challengers brought new ideas and practices into childbirth, and they are still on the stage; later we will return to their new tactics in institutionalized care. Since then, many new actors – not only independent midwives but also a broad range of birth attendants, from doulas (Ozhiganova, 2021) to perinatal psychologists – have appeared in post-Soviet maternity care, and they all produce their own ideas of "good care" (see Chapter 4).

In this section, we address the ways in which midwives are initiating some alterations within formal, mainstream institutions, thereby improving the quality of maternity care. We argue that personal leadership, communicative skills, recruitment of supporters and new ideas comprise the opportunities for some changes in maternity institutions to happen. Other scholars (Borozdina, 2014b, 2017, 2018; Borozdina & Novkunskaya, 2020) have described cases in which midwives have initiated changes in maternity hospitals in post-Soviet Russia. For example, a unique special center (ward) for midwifery care, called "Rainbow," emerged in St. Petersburg in 1997 as a commercial department in a State-funded maternity hospital, where several midwives, supported by a few obstetricians and the chief, tried to develop an approach oriented toward "natural" and women-centered childbirth (Borozdina, 2014b, 2017, 2018). The initial ideas for this department came from the homebirth movement and from some Russian midwives who undertook international training (Borozdina & Novkunskaya, 2020). Continuity and personalization of midwifery care were the key principles underlying maternity services in this department; these were quite different from the State-funded conveyer-like principle, which led to depersonalization and fragmentation of maternity care (see Chapter 3). According to the new principles in the Rainbow center, every childbearing woman was recommended to prepare for childbirth in advance and to choose a certain midwife who would personally monitor her pregnancy and assist her in labor and birth. An obstetrician would intervene only if deemed necessary by the midwife; this was informally agreed upon in the hospital, though legally the ultimate responsibility for the results was still held by an obstetrician, not by the midwife who provided the entire range of maternity care. Women's partners were encouraged to actively participate in childbirth, and new techniques and comfort conditions were introduced in the labor ward. After the maternity hospital in which these midwives were located was closed in the 2010s, they tried to find new locations in other hospitals, and finally, in two maternity hospitals, they now provide support to women with "individual contracts." Activists are working to maintain "Rainbow" practices as centers for women who want to receive support from midwives, though the status of such initiatives is uncertain.

Some other cases are described by social researchers in which midwives are relatively autonomous and can challenge the conditions of maternity care provision or professional approaches to childbirth within their maternity units. In these cases, midwives play more equal roles with obstetricians, comprising a team oriented toward the new, more women-friendly, and less medicalized approach. Sometimes such midwives even achieve a quasi-independent practice in which the midwife assists a woman on her own, if there are no identifiable risks (Novkunskaya, 2018; Ozhiganova, 2020; Borozdina & Novkunskaya, 2020).

Thus, midwifery agency and holistic approaches in such niches of maternity care are developing. However, such initiatives, accomplished as the innovative institutional work of midwives (Borozdina, 2018), achieve limited spread and recognition. Although relatively successful in some communities or localities, they have never received mass support among maternity care providers nor among care receivers and their families. These cases of changes in maternity care are rare and exceptional and do not take a systemic character, as they do not shape nor challenge the System on a larger scale.

More examples are given by Anna Ozhiganova (2019b, 2021) of semi-informal negotiations and agreements made within maternity hospitals, in which independent, homebirth midwives or doulas achieve formal affiliation with some hospitals, and consequently the opportunity to provide labor support to their clients even within institutionalized settings. Again, in such centers, childbirth cannot be legally attended; officially, these centers only prepare women for hospital birth. Semi-informal possibilities have been opened for challengers: some independent midwifery centers opted to make official commercial contracts with maternity hospitals, and then midwives could come to the hospital with their clients and support them during labor and birth. Other midwives or "independent" maternity care providers who had medical education in their backgrounds – which became popular for independent midwives to receive starting in the mid-2000s (Ozhiganova, 2021) – obtained official positions in hospitals and received formal rights to support women in hospital delivery. Doulas providing non-medical support also became allowed to attend hospital-based births as women's officially permitted "partners." Their positions and opportunities to provide labor support depend on informal relationships with providers in a given hospital (Ozhiganova, 2021). Maternity hospitals have a financial interest in attracting more clients, and thus invest in advertising "natural," "soft" delivery or quasi-homebirth settings as paid-for services, which promise better conditions, personalized care, limited medicalization and emotional support (by doulas). However, doulas' official status remains unclear, their participation is far from being non-problematic, and they may be denied in access to hospitals, as many hospital midwives, obstetricians and chiefs are unfriendly toward any "alternative" practices. Moreover, competition for clients emerges between those who promote new approaches – doulas, independent midwives and some hospital practitioners.

Hospital midwives struggling for "good care": from informalities to professional associations

As our empirical data show (see Appendix 1), the set of reforms introduced into healthcare and medical education since the 2010s produced a new type of agents in the maternity care field. Along with other authors, we argue that midwives' leadership, informal professional relationships, constant personal negotiations and teamwork have been key resources employed to make comprehensive changes in maternity care. Autonomous professional midwifery associations did not exist in Soviet society, but since the mid-1990s, some transformations were initiated in official (State-related) associations, and in the early 2000s, some midwifery activities developed within nursing associations. On the official level, these changes included increasing international communications, organizing conferences and developing collaborations with different regions. In the 2010s, sections of midwives within nursing associations appeared, and even some Soviet successors have transformed into creating more favorable spaces for professional discussions among maternity and health care providers. Yet, as challengers complain, conference participants prefer to report about their successes, and not to voice practical problems and actual needs of midwives or patients.

Some actors have started to challenge the existing rules of highly medicalized birth, the total subordination of midwives and nurses to obstetricians, the silencing of their public voices and the absence of legal responsibilities (independent midwifery is illegal; obstetricians are legally responsible for childbirth and must always be present). Professional associations of midwives have tried to support some new initiatives (such as "Rainbow"), find empowering contacts within the international community, mobilize midwives and promote changes in education, such as a new system of ongoing recertification of nurses and midwives.[1] However, these are concerns of only a small circle of challengers. On the official level, associations try to establish contacts with authorities, though they say that they must struggle to be heard. But their voices can barely challenge top-down recommendations and decisions on work or education in midwifery and nursing.

According to our midwife interlocutors, who are active and take leadership positions within associations, hospitals and educational systems, their first ideas for changes often emerged from their own childbirth experiences. They invoked some cases when something was going wrong, when they tried to achieve some alternative conditions for their own births, or they were not satisfied with the services provided in maternity hospitals. Such experiences inspired them to seek changes. Gradually, from their first attempts to articulate and deal with the problem, they recognized its root as "*the System, where is nobody is interested in a woman and a newborn*" (focus group).

Their next steps were meeting with like-minded colleagues ("*supporters*") and generating new ideas about childbirth and midwifery. Ideas for change often come from other colleagues, especially from those who have connections with practitioners from other countries, who could share their experiences of more humanized birth practices. Some international cooperation has indeed developed between professional associations; sometimes these too have been personal, informal contacts with relatives, friends or colleagues involved in maternity care abroad.

Those midwives who have become challengers have undertaken additional nursing higher education to obtain a Master's degree; they continue to make many efforts to self-educate and to communicate with those who practice "natural" childbirth (less medicalized and more autonomous). However, our midwife interlocutors say that even today, ideas about independent midwives working in maternity hospitals remain irrelevant and unpopular; there is no interest at the rank-and-file incumbent level; and obstetricians are opposed to such ideas, or do not take them seriously.

Challengers from midwives' associations have been organizing special sessions at obstetric-gynecological conferences since the 2010s, and nursing associations also have their own regular official workshops, but these are mostly only spaces for formal presentations without discussions, or for official celebrations, with no voice for those who want changes. However, at the same time, some informal talks or clubs developed ("*shifts with secret supporters in the night*" – from a focus group), in which midwives discussed less medicalized approaches to childbirth, negotiated more freedom for women, less regulated processes and more authority and autonomy for midwives. At that time, such ideas were, according to our interlocutors, rather provocative and were not discussed publicly. They named themselves "*partisans*," secretly discussing Michel Odent, "spiritual midwifery," and other "forbidden" topics. Their activities on the ground level have been important for consciousness raising.

Such challengers appeal to the international, like-minded professional community, and our interlocutors refer to the authentically Russian practice of water birth – which originated in Russia due to the work of Igor Charkovsky (see Belooussova, 2002; Ozhiganova, 2019c), but was popularized worldwide by obstetrician Michel Odent (Odent, 1984); "hypno-birthing"; or "prophylactic psychological prevention (of mental and health disorders)," as some midwives call it. At the same time, ideas about "natural" childbirth became popular, and many obstetricians in commercial departments became ready to meet some of these demands (Borozdina, 2014b).

From the mid-2010s to the present, some challengers started to vocalize the need for institutional changes in medical education, midwifery and nursing research, and the improvement of hand-on practices. They also stand for more professional autonomy for midwives and right to deal with physiological pregnancies independently, arguing that women will be more satisfied and receive better care, and obstetricians will be less overburdened. Their activities have become more public; they present their ideas in workshops and conferences and comment with irony that, only a few years ago, it was possible to discuss such issues only in their kitchens (i.e., informally). One response from a colleague in one of our focus group discussions was:

> *I liked it so much! That is so cool! I can't even believe it! You stand in this pulpit, say it out loud! Not somewhere out there . . . where no one can see, in the kitchen. You talk about it out loud at the conference!*

Professional associations try to get more influence on new professional and educational standards; they manage to mobilize support in maternity hospitals for changes, and some nurses, midwives and obstetricians support them, yet evaluate their overall influences as very slight.

When we asked how professional associations manage to mobilize resources and support for certain changes, their representatives explained this by their "charisma" and their persistent, endless efforts, which sometimes are very emotional in discussions and other communications. For example, in order to receive a document she needed, one midwife made 19 (stress with a voice in her narrative: *nineteen!*) telephone calls. Leadership, personal involvement and imbuing the incumbents with new ideas are crucial for those midwives "*who are concerned and want to do something*" (interview with an association official).

Their goals are moderate, and not political per se – with the exception of the COVID-19 period, when they were ready to become more explicitly political, as practitioners received little support from the State and had problems in obtaining personal protective equipment (PPE) and precise clinical recommendations. Associations mobilized their social and professional networks to attract resources (financial, administrative) and spread cutting-edge international recommendations, both formally and informally. Thus, many COVID-related problems were solved to some extent without direct political actions. But this grassroots mobilization appeared to be an important example of effectiveness of joint actions and professional solidarity. Along with such wide-scale actions, challengers break the stalemate – from "partisans" they turn into the avant-garde of their professional groups (nurses and midwives). In addition to their strategy of local changes (in their own ward or in hospitals), they struggle for the right to challenge the System.

Such challengers mobilize support for their initiatives from different medical professionals and try to communicate them to nurses, physicians and bureaucrats, including those who are not very supportive of their initiatives. These activists are oriented toward legal changes, and thus try to influence the State bodies; however, often they receive no reaction for years. Some influence can be obtained via tactics of mobilization of informal networks, "telephone law," and administrative resources (a kind of manual management). They complain that these bodies often prefer to ignore them and to pretend that the problems require different solutions or already effectively addressed. One midwife describes these relationships with the State (the System) using the following metaphor:

> *The System put me in a cage. I'm a hostage. System says: "Don't stick your head out! Do you understand?" I say: "I understand, but I will try and continue." The System says: "Well, then blame yourself!" You will do it somehow, somehow! But there will be no support for this.*
>
> *(focus group, midwife)*

Positive changes within a single hospital seem to be a success, but now challengers are aware that there is a need and potential for more scaled transformations. But incumbents remain a serious obstacle – there is no "critical mass" of those ready to vocalize their dissatisfaction, resources are still limited, and the System is not responsive. Rank-and-file (incumbent) professionals are often suspicious of new approaches and of significant transformations in maternity care provision and professional education, afraid of threats to their stability. They are also suspicious of associations and any official organizations, asking "*For what do I need this membership? What will this association give to me?*" (interview with a midwife). Midwives are overburdened, mostly working in maternity hospitals in 24-hour shifts and additionally in commercial departments. Obstetricians and chiefs are often far from understanding the advantages of changes promoted by midwives/challengers and are afraid that they could shatter their own (usually already vulnerable) positions.

As subalterns, midwives doubt that they can speak and be heard; thus, struggling with the System is limited to only a few hospital midwife enthusiasts who work to inspire their colleagues. However, hospital midwives now also recognize that their voices can be heard, and, as a result, many of those who used to be strongly opposed to more women-friendly approaches and a plurality of techniques now adopt these innovations in their own practices. The concept of "supporting women in childbirth" has been put into action in various practices, and communication has become more important in relations between care providers and care receivers. The quality of care consequently gradually changes; more variety has become acceptable, at least in commercial departments; and now women can arrive with their birth plans and those plans will be taken into account – quite a significant change. Challengers use the tactic of "small steps," and they say that this is a female (sometimes feminist) way of struggle. They hope that Russian midwives will ultimately comprise an autonomous profession, oriented toward continuity of care and improving the quality of care, so that women will be more satisfied with their birth experiences and more empowered by those experiences. For this to happen, first of all, the system of midwifery education must be changed in ways that prepare midwives for independent work, research, critical thinking, person-oriented communication, continuity of care and more personalized care.

Activists and an independent trade union struggling for "good care": public voices and the case of Hospital M.

Here we present the case of one maternity care department in a remote area (for details, see Appendix 1), in which practitioners protested against top-down reforms, mobilizing the support of the public, the media and an independent trade union. These practitioners as challengers acted strategically and politically, fighting for their professional rights and patients' safety. First, we describe the context and the story of this protest, and then we focus on its strategies of struggle.

The context of this case is framed by recent reforms that have led to a decline in the number of maternity care units in the country (see Chapter 3): the maternity care hospitals or departments are marketized and forced to earn money, but, being unable to introduce paid services, are often appear to be unprofitable. The so-called "optimization" of services more directly affects remote and small Level 1 maternity facilities (Novkunskaya, 2020), resulting in the elimination of practitioners' positions and the worsening of maternity care accessibility for the women living in such areas. Such decisions, as a rule, are made by regional authorities, carried out by hospital administrators and are often met with extreme resistance on the parts of maternity care providers and receivers, whose responses sometimes take the forms of strategic and political protests.

The particular maternity care department that we describe here is located in Hospital M., which is in one of the district centers of Central Russia and used to be a Level 2 facility; until 2016, it assisted around 800–900 births per year. Over the past few years, this department has undergone institutional reformation, including a reduction in the number of its beds and of its maternity care providers, and its re-assignment as a Level 1 facility with lower capacities. Such reforms caused discontent and the mobilization of the maternity care providers in this department in alliance with the independent trade union of medical practitioners.

Maternity Hospital M. is located 110 km from the capital, in a city with 30,000 residents. Its facilities are also available to residents of the entire district – more than 70,000 people living in an area of 27,000 square kilometers – and to the residents of two neighboring regions. Until recently, the maternity hospital itself (administratively, a maternity department of the M. Central District Hospital), was located in a five-storey building constructed in the late Soviet period, and occupied all five floors. Until 2017, before this maternity hospital was demoted to Level 1, it could accept pregnant women with pathologies, and with certain pregnancy risks and complications, as it had intensive care wards for mothers and newborns, the round-the-clock presence of an obstetrician-gynecologist, a neonatologist, midwives and nurses.

At the end of 2016, the situation changed. A new Level 3 perinatal center was opened in the region, more than 85 kilometers from the Hospital M.; this rearranged the routing of pregnant women, as the most complicated pregnancies were now to be directed to the new perinatal center. This new routing scheme assumed reducing the number of childbirths in Hospital M., and resulted in the economic "optimization" of its capacity and number of providers in 2017. This caused a "rebellion," as participants called it. In an interview, one of the most active midwives of the case described this rebellion as follows:

> *We [in 2017] already understood what was happening then and began to rebel, as we say, I don't know how else to express it. We then began to be indignant: "what was happening?!" The staff of the maternity hospital was cut – not in half, most of it, a lot! If in a shift we used to have up to 4–5 midwives, then there remained – after this "optimization" – just 1.5-1 [per shift]!*
>
> (interview with Hospital M. midwife)

The whole building, designed for 60 inpatient maternity beds, which had been recently renovated and had purchased expensive medical equipment, was reorganized: the maternity department was merged with the gynecological department and left to be located only on two floors of the renovated building, and only seven midwives remained on the staff, so in some shifts there was only one midwife left for all wards. This not only led to an increase in the burden on these midwives but also increased the risks for pregnant and birthing women. This "optimization" took place under the formal reasoning that the level and status of Hospital M. had been changed; it now was prescribed to provide only basic maternity services and assist with only uncomplicated childbirths, while all the rest of the pregnancies had to be routed to the new perinatal center.

Outraged residents and employees of this maternity unit asked to meet at a round table, with the participation of representatives of the new perinatal center, the staff of the maternity hospital, and representatives of some public organizations acting in the district, and also organized an open event with the participation of State Duma deputies and journalists to answer questions from the district residents. The head physician of the M. Central Hospital explained why he could not sustain the maternity department's previous status, although all other departments of the Central Hospital remained within the Level 2 status: there was no money for this:

> *Now to maintain such a department [of the second level], I, as a head, on whose shoulders lies a huge financial burden, I cannot 'feed' it – I apologize for this expression!*
>
> *(video with the head physician of the M. Central District Hospital)*

Another problem emerged, this time over transportation. According to a midwife of the maternity department of Hospital M., improved transport infrastructure should be developed between the maternity department of M. and the new perinatal center. The chief of the perinatal center promised to organize a daily bus for those medical practitioners who were forced to work in the new perinatal center, that is, every day to travel 85 kilometers in one direction, and then return home. In addition, special regular transport had to be organized for pregnant women for necessary services, as ultrasound and other types of screening were transferred to the perinatal center. In addition, the ambulance services, which are responsible for patient transportation, are not integrated into the hospitals' network. Paramedics of the ambulance opt to drive women to the nearest maternity unit, and they sometimes still transfer women with risky pregnancies to the M. maternity unit, which cannot officially assist in such cases and is no longer sufficiently equipped for them. All this provoked participants' discontent; they received promises from the administration, but no real support or action.

The working conditions for maternity care providers across the country became more challenging at the beginning of the coronavirus pandemic in early March 2020. In the spring of 2020, with the increase in the cases of COVID-19, the maternity department of Hospital M. was reorganized into a COVID treatment department. The maternity department moved to just two wards of the surgical department and was prescribed to take only emergency cases, while routine maternity care was no longer provided there. The positions of pediatric and gynecological nurses were liquidated, and these nurses were asked to look for new jobs on their own. At the time of the pandemic, only midwives were left in the department – one for a day shift: in addition to her usual duties, this midwife had to register and examine the arriving women, and to provide the operating table (which used to be a function of the surgery nurse) if a woman came with bleeding, and then to wash the floor as well, because the department did not have its own attendants or cleaners. In addition, PPE was not supplied, as maternity care practitioners were not formally supposed to be exposed to the COVID-19 infected patients, and, hence, if they nevertheless met, they had to find PPE on their own. Under all these critical conditions, in 2020, the maternity department's practitioners joined the independent trade union "Alliance of Physicians" in order to fight for their labor rights, and this was an important step in their struggle, to which we later return.

After the first wave of COVID-19 cases, the maternity department returned to former floors, but then, within two months, the second wave began and the department had to move again, this time to the fifth floor in the therapeutic building in the former gynecological department. In May 2021, inspection by Rospotrebnadzor made the prescription that the maternity department could no longer accept even emergency deliveries, since the new location does not meet sanitary standards and requirements: for example, the special kitchen for milk is not equipped. All women in labor had to be taken to the perinatal center by ambulance.

Women were confused by these re-organizations of maternity care. In 2017–2018, the maternity hospital in the neighboring district R. was closed in the course of the same "optimization." During this second wave, one woman came to M. from this region in her personal car; she did not know that the maternity hospital had been ordered not to assist deliveries. This woman entered the emergency room of the therapeutic department, whose practitioners never even checked cervical dilation, but called their colleagues from the gynecological (former maternity) department:

> *We came running from the fifth floor, and the newborn's head was almost visible – where [could we] take her? The woman was quickly taken to the fifth floor, she gave birth there just in the exam room, although we had no right to assist with birth! The ambulance, which at that time was working for COVID-19 and was loaded with cases of*

> *infection, was able to arrive only 5 hours after the delivery. Since the department's nurses were laid off and there is no neonatologist now, the newborn could not get necessary help during all this time, because [I as a] midwife am limited by a certificate – I cannot approach him!*
>
> (Interview with Hospital M. midwife)

Simultaneously with the official prescriptions of Rospotrebnadzor, a new wave of personnel cuts began: in April 2021, the chief physician of the M. Central Hospital notified his employees about the upcoming reduction from 16 June 2021, according to which there will be a further reduction of beds in the maternity department. And this has caused more discontent.

A collision developed among the top incumbents – the hospital administration and the perinatal center, regional authorities, other government bodies and healthcare managers from the top, and the challengers from below – maternity care providers – midwives, nurses and obstetricians-gynecologists. These challengers are currently resisting such reforms and trying to maintain the former structure of maternity care. This is both strategic and political action as they try to take control over the situation in opposition to the incumbents, who simply follow the path of top-down reforms.

At the first stage of the reorganization, the practitioners of maternity Hospital M. appealed to the public – a relatively rare strategy in Russia. They initiated public discussions of the current situation with regional and federal deputies, local media and public organizations. This strategy did not lead to success, the promises made by healthcare managers were not fulfilled and the reconstruction and reduction continued. In 2020, the practitioners opted for a new strategy: they reached out to the independent professional union "Alliance of Physicians" for legal and media support, and in doing so, their public voice became noticeable.

As background and context, here we briefly clarify the situation of this trade union. Official trade unions in Russian healthcare (and in general) are of a particular type, mostly having a Soviet legacy. In Soviet medicine, trade unions did not perform the function of real struggle for labor interests, yet played an important symbolic role associated with the rhetoric of the "dictatorship of the proletariat," and were used to working as State regulative bodies. They dealt with politically insignificant local problems related to public welfare, such as the distribution of vouchers to sanatoriums (health resorts for employers, employees and their families), and the organization of so-called "socialist competition" among practitioners as socialist workers for better results (in statistical indicators) of their work. Currently, such "pocket" (i.e., close to hospital administrations, as if "in their pockets") trade unions perform similar functions – the distribution of small resources such as vouchers and the organization of holidays.

The Alliance of Physicians, founded in 2018, is quite a different type of organization – a relatively new independent trade union, which, according to the official information on its website, has offices in 42 regions of Russia and several thousand members. It was founded by ophthalmologist Anastasia Vasilyeva, who fought to maintain her department in the course of "optimization" and, being personally acquainted with Alexei Navalny, one of the most famous opposition politicians in Russia, adopted the strategies of political struggle, transferring them to the professional field of medical care. Later, she was forced to leave her department and became an independent trade union official.

Social and political closeness with opposition to power structures, as well as similar strategies used – media coverage of various controversial situations and an attempt to resolve them in the legal field – initially marked the activities of the Alliance of Physicians as political. In 2021, the Ministry of Justice registered the organization on the list of so-called "Foreign Agents" – a labeling indicating that NGOs receive money from sources outside the Russian Federation. As the website of the trade union signifies, the organization does not agree with the Ministry of Justice and considers assignment to this status as unfair. This position of the trade union is a marker of the politicization of professional work in Russian biomedicine. According to the Law on Foreign Agents, this status is also assigned to those organizations that are engaged in "political activity," which means that the work of the union of medical allies is officially recognized as political. The representative of the trade union did not deny this state of affairs – in his opinion, medicine in Russia is by default a field of political actions:

> *And you want to say that medicine is possible without politics? I do not believe in this. This does not happen . . . in any country, especially in ours, healthcare is a hyper-regulated area. In our country, all regulation in healthcare is based on the State institutions. Starting from Roszdravnadzor, ending . . . with Rostekhnadzor [Russian Technical Surveillance]. Yes.*
>
> (interview with deputy chairman of the trade union "Alliance of Physicians")

"The political" here is understood not only as the status of a (political) "Foreign Agent" but also as a high degree of State political involvement in the practical work of medicine and healthcare. With the support of this union, which is defined by activists as *enlightenment* (as one midwife said, "*Thanks to them, we understand more about what's going on*"), strategies undertaken by the maternity care practitioners of Hospital M. have expanded. A midwife working in this hospital described the repertoire of their political actions; after other actions did not bring results, they wrote petitions and declared an "Italian strike":

> *We have already found ourselves at the end of our rope – we have contacted the [Ministry of] healthcare, we have contacted Roszdravnadzor, we went to the Presidential Administration, we wrote a letter to the President . . . [but] we have all these gears of the government moving very slowly, . . . and here again we cannot calm down – we see no justice, we have reached the point where we declared an Italian strike. When we declared the Italian strike, we ourselves were frightened [of these words] – for us it is scary, we are people of the Soviet type. We are working, and [suddenly] we receive a call from the hospital administration: "Has everyone come to work? Isn't anyone skipping?" Later we caught up with the fact that the administration was not aware of what the Italian strike was – that it was just work in accordance with our labor contracts, without fulfilling additional obligations.*
>
> (interview with midwife of Hospital M.)

As this midwife states, the hospital administration does not understand the meaning of the "Italian strike"; medical practitioners are scared, do not always have a good understanding of their labor rights, and can use illegal actions in their strategies. Thus, the very articulation of such violations becomes a political act. The Alliance of Physicians, on behalf of their members from the maternity department of the Hospital M., expanded their repertoire of strategic actions by issuing a petition on the *change.org* website describing the situation around the M. maternity hospital and calling to stop the reduction and return it to its former Level 2 status. In three months, the petition collected more than 30,000 signatures. Another strategy was to increase the visibility of the problem by increasing its media coverage: as the trade union representative explained, "*Yes, this is a deliberate strategy [publishing in the media]. We are sincere. We have a principle that publicity is our weapon!*"

The case of Hospital M. demonstrates the inconsistency of State representation and regulation. Besides belonging to the independent trade union, all other participants are either State employees or State representatives (see also Chapter 3): the field as a whole is State-related. "State" can be a confusing concept, though it is mostly referred as "The State" – "a supervisory club" that overregulates and controls maternity care provision in unnecessary and inconsistent ways, as the deputy chairman of the independent trade union explained:

> *Again, we have all these things, all these orders – they are regulated by the legislative, not even legislative, you know, such a supervisory club. That is, the more the powerful the "club". . . that interferes with*

> *a medical organization and controls it, the more effectively it is considered to work according to their laws.*
>
> (interview with deputy chairman of the trade union "Alliance of Physicians")

Different actors in this field define in different ways the goals and objectives of their actions, and consequently, what constitutes "good care" for them. For multiple controlling and supervisory bodies, "good care" is the fulfillment of all existing formal orders and standards for each department. For healthcare managers and hospital administration, "good care" consists of the effectiveness of maternity care provision in terms of economic feasibility:

> *But, unfortunately, with us, you perfectly understand that [in our system] the main person in the hospital is the head physician. The head physician has his own economic interests, well, they understand economic interests very wrongly, unfortunately, nothing can be done about this in our country. . . . How exactly? Well, I've already talked about saving . . . The ideal chief physician is a doctor who, let's say, can get as much money from the organization as possible.*
>
> (interview with deputy chairman of the trade union "Alliance of Physicians")

And although the study participants also mentioned corruption, we are talking here about the legal and economic rationales regarding the entire work of the institution, Hospital M. The maternity ward was not economically profitable, and this ultimately became the reason for its termination.

For maternity care providers and care receivers, "good care" is connected to the maternity hospital as a place of sizable numbers of qualified practitioners, and as a place that guarantees safety and good service for childbearing women. These participants are also fighting for their voices to be heard and for autonomy in their positions, describing these desires via a metaphor of how the paths in a park should be laid in a rational way based on real practices and on the voices of "real people":

> *There is no need to decide the fate of people in offices! We must solve them on the spot! You have to ask people! You just listen to people – what people need – people will lay paths where they are comfortable. And before you make stone paths, look where they have already been trodden! And lay these sidewalks in the same place. You listen to people and find out what they need! But no one in our country listens to people, everything is decided at the top.*
>
> (interview with Hospital M. midwife)

Participants critically and metaphorically define the System they oppose as *a concrete wall*, within which they feel themselves as slaves (as in the description in the previous section of a *hostage in a cage*). The maternity care practitioners of Hospital M., who had quite limited resources to keep their maternity unit stable and functioning, described all the changes that have taken place as imposed from the top-down and insensitive to the local conditions, rank-and-file initiatives and the practices of those who provided and received services in Hospital M. It turns out that strategic actions in this case were aimed at the empowerment of maternity care providers, on the one hand, and at achieving the conditions that are necessary for "good care," on the other. This is how an obstetrician-gynecologist of the M. maternity hospital described the ultimate goal of all this activity in a media publication:

> *Now I have written a report, tomorrow I will go to the head of our city, because it is impossible when a doctor does not even have the ability to provide assistance to a patient . . . The correctness of the modernization and everything else [reforms] will be assessed later on. The main thing for me is that in my city, where women, my relatives, my children live, there are vital medical services. We do not need high-tech help, [in complicated cases] we will go to neighboring cities for it, thank God, there are [necessary services]. But we need the most necessary things here.*
>
> (media publication, interview with obstetrician-gynecologist of the M. maternity hospital)

To conclude our lengthy discussion of the case of Hospital M., we note that the strategic actions taken by multiple challengers have not achieved the desired results: the maternity ward remains closed, women still cannot give birth in this area, and some of the employees have been forced to find new jobs outside of the hospital and even of the district in which they have built their lives and those of their families. However, the set of actions taken constitutes a vivid example of the commitment of a professional group to the ideals of "good care," which inspired them to start a strategic/political struggle even without having sufficient resources and remaining a part of a State-regulated field. Here we stress the differences between activities in the central cities that are fused with commercialization in their innovations (which are mostly responses to clients' requests) and the more openly political actions taken by overt challengers in this remote area of the country.

Some of the ideals and practices of "good care" emerge in the marginal areas of maternity care, and then are spread to a wider number of situations. The current status quo in maternity care is challenged by those actors who help to make care more women-oriented and empowering to them, especially in situations of reproductive loss, as we describe in the following section.

NGOs struggling for "good care": the case of perinatal palliative care

Philanthropy in the sphere of maternity care includes NGOs (non-governmental organizations) that provide support for families who face various struggles related to peri- and postnatal period. The list of services provided by such NGOs usually includes psychological help, emotional and informational support and medical and financial aid for those families who need it. These could be those experience reproductive loss (miscarriage, stillbirth, abortion for a medical reason); whose newborns were diagnosed with incurable diseases; who delivered premature babies or babies with rare clinical conditions; low-resource families; etc. Some of the NGOs are co-sponsored by the State – for instance, they can receive funds by winning governmental grant competitions – or depend on private donations. The scale of changes provided by these organizations has a broad domain – from low-budget groups of enthusiasts to technologically equipped units with high-skilled professionals. In this section, we analyze one of such organizations, which is *challenging* the current approaches to working with women in vulnerable situations of unfavorable prognosis for unborn (for more details on data, see Appendix 1) – a perinatal palliative care program run by a charity foundation.

Institutionally, the care of the unborn is shared between several actors on different levels: the State, maternity care providers, and women. All of them have their own ideas about what constitutes "good care." The unborn possesses a precarious position (Hockey & Draper, 2005; Keane, 2009) and therefore is attributed socio-cultural meaning, depending on the context (Layne, 2003, p. 240; Keane, 2009, p. 157). Generally, reproductive loss involves the interaction of numerous actors (women, medical personnel, psychologists, family members) who are actively involved in the discursive and material production of meanings, but whose interpretations/positions of the situation may differ significantly. The institutional meanings of loss, which are formed in the process of institutional interactions, often do not correspond to women's perceptions, thereby causing additional suffering. Women articulate the highest degrees of suffering as occurring in situations in which they were treated with rudeness (*khamstvo*) from maternity care practitioners, were not permitted to see and touch their stillborn babies, and experienced unwanted respond to their emotions ("*Stop crying!*" "*It was not a baby yet!*").

Nowadays, as previously noted, Russian women's discontent with maternity care, particularly in situations of reproductive loss, is becoming more articulated. Grassroots initiatives such as support groups, and particular specialists (e.g., psychologists working with perinatal loss), have emerged. Over time, some of these initiatives have taken institutionalized forms – they stem into charitable foundations and educational projects, one of which we will provide as an example of such initiatives later.

At the moment, a large number of experts are participating in the discussion about reproductive loss. Previously, the discourses around reproductive losses were monopolized by obstetricians-gynecologists, who reduced such losses almost exclusively to their medical aspects. Now, more and more expert communities are involved – medical care providers (obstetricians-gynecologists, midwives, specialists in ultrasound diagnostics and palliative care), psychologists, employees of charitable organizations, helping professionals such as doulas and "lay experts" such as women with their own experiences of loss.

Activists of NGOs that have appeared relatively recently try to fill the gaps and to provide women with care they cannot receive in existing State-funded institutions. Their projects and activism stem from their personal experiences, which revealed the gaps in care provision for such women, and respond to increasing requests from women searching for relevant help and telling their stories of *khamstvo* and aggression during miscarriage, stillbirth or death of a newborn in the neonatal intensive care unit (NICU). Women articulate their needs to stay with a dying newborn, permission to touch and care, make some memorial rituals, remain with the body for a time (in most birth rooms and NICUs, all these actions are forbidden) and, most importantly, to not be treated rudely by providers (*khamstvo*).

One such NGO provides a perinatal palliative care service working on the basis of hospice care for children. Its aim is to provide help to women and families who are expecting the birth of an incurable child. Such hospice activist practitioners are ready to provide information, psychological help and emotional support and to organize advanced home-based care for those whose babies are born alive but require palliative support (lung ventilation, special ways of feeding, etc.). This palliative care program, launched in 2018, is the first of its kind in Russia and is working only in Moscow and its immediate surroundings.

This perinatal palliative service is organized as follows. A childbearing woman in Moscow, whose unborn has been diagnosed with a severe malformation, is routed to the city *consilium* – experts of different medical specializations (genetics, psychologists, neonatologists, etc.) who are to confirm the prognosis and give recommendations. If the prognosis remains unfavorable, this NGO offers the family participation in its perinatal palliative program. In such a case, the childbirth will take place in a certain maternity hospital, and during pregnancy, labor, birth and the postnatal period, the woman will receive special services, such as training courses for stillbirth or for the birth of a baby who will soon die, information on legal and medical issues, psychological consultations, the possibility to memorialize the child (make casts of the baby, have professional photos taken, spend time with the baby in a special farewell room, baptize a child right in the birth room, etc.), and the provision of needed medical devices for taking a palliative infant home.

This perinatal palliative care program includes a neonatologist, an obstetrician, a psychologist, a photographer and others. Behind and supportive of this small group, there is a larger team of obstetricians, midwives, and neonatologists from the maternity hospital in which the program is realized. The implementation of these new ideas and practices is not always easy, but is exactly how this NGO challenges the System. By now, this program is ready to offer help to all who need it in Moscow. The program works as a pilot project and therefore cannot yet be spread to other regions. But it challenges the existing practices and ideas of "good care."

Before this program started, parents were to write to the children's hospice, explaining that they were expecting a dead or extremely ill baby and asking for help and advice – but there was nothing to offer them. Parents who gave birth to babies with incurable diseases narrated their stories of experiencing *khamstvo* during pregnancy, labor, and birth, and/or in the postnatal period, and that their practitioners tried to persuade them not to prolong the pregnancy or not to take a sick baby home. After birth, such a baby usually is taken to the NICU, and parents can visit their babies for a very limited time per day, they cannot touch or hold their baby, and sometimes are not allowed to take the body to be buried. In such cases, personal emotions intertwine with professional agency. Their stories caused a group of enthusiasts in the children's hospice NGO to start the program. Many interlocutors referred to the book written by Anna Starobinets (2017) about her experiences of perinatal loss and unconcerned maternity care practitioners, which became a bestseller in Russia. They wanted to challenge the System; as this NGO program developed full-scale, its originators mobilized various actors – parents who wanted changes, physicians (chief specialists in neonatology and palliative care) and high-ranking officials:

> *And in May 2017, I guess, we – such positive and active people – have written that we now have perinatal palliative care. [Speaks ironically.] That's all. We didn't know what to do next and where to look for all those pregnant women. Well, [our hospice director] wrote a post in her Facebook, but nobody connected with us . . . At the same time, we didn't understand in detail what to do. Well, we wrote here and there – and got silence back. And in November 2018, the first patient appealed to us, and we started this way together with her. And I must also say that this was the time when Nyuta Federmesser [a co-founder of the fund and well-known charity leader] asked the mayor of the city to do something for the development of perinatal palliative care in Moscow. And he produced an order to make a pilot project . . . and addressed its realization to several perinatal centers. But there is no need to list them, because only one took part in its realization.*
>
> (interview with the head of the NGO palliative care service)

Activists working in this NGO were ready to implement their project, and as in the case of midwives, a lot of small steps were needed, such as to recruit committed participants and to find allies and resources. For large-scale changes, they needed a political will that would get their recommendations authorized, but decisions from "the top" were crucial:

> *And perinatal [palliative] care – it appeared because you notice a baby and understand that help is needed, but there is no help . . . You start to move. But this is very hard . . . It is important that several issues matched: a competent person appeared – the one who wants to do that, there was a demand, and there was a decision from the top, right?. . . That is there is demand, manager and "you are welcome" – and go ahead, you have the green light. In Moscow in perinatal [palliative] care, we now have it.*
>
> (interview with Nyuta Federmesser, co-founder of the charity fund)

NGOs try to find resources and supporters in the ruling bodies and professional organizations who could become their allies in the promotion and provision of changes in institutional women's support: obstetricians and midwives who seek to challenge the current principles of care, as well as State officials interested in the organizational and financial benefits of such changes. To become sustainable, NGOs try to build networks of people who share the same ideals of "good care" and to attract resources (administrative, financial, professional) to put them into practice. NGOs receive financing from donations and grants (including some provided by the State). They also get substantial help from volunteers, who offer their professional help pro bono (provide psychological consultations, take photographs, etc.) or help with the daily routines (answer calls, help with transportation, etc.). In some special cases, the government can also subsidize certain needs of significant organizations – for instance, it covers 20% of the expenses of this charity foundation, which has several programs, including the children's hospice and perinatal palliative care programs.

This NGO's efforts to challenge the System face resistance from the incumbents who want to preserve the existing order. Changing the extant rules is an uneasy task, as, again, incumbents are suspicious about new agents and new rules; they are afraid of destabilizing existing institutions and of extra burdens and duties, as they already feel vulnerable and overburdened:

> *But, frankly speaking, midwives do not like to be bothered with antenatal [deaths] . . . There will be smell, and appearance, and all that . . . Well, because there can be some really disfiguring forms [of malformations] . . . Well, they don't have time for it either, indeed.*
>
> (interview with clinical psychologist, pediatrician, works at NGO)

Given that the field of maternity care is highly medicalized and subordinated to State bodies, it is very important for challengers to establish personal relationships with officials in governance units, and to mobilize administrative resources. They point at the flaws in governmental implementations of "good care" and demonstrate its inefficacy. But they also offer solutions and mobilize resources that are absent in State-funded health and maternity care institutions to improve the situation; they bring best practices that increase women's satisfaction with the provision of maternity care. NGOs help the System by organizing care in the niches and gaps that cannot be filled in otherwise, due to financial or organizational challenges:

> *I mean, talking with parents, for instance, about the way a baby will die, what we will do then, what we will do after the baby's death, whether we will take the body to bury or not. Nobody except us is ready to talk about this with parents. That's why – yes – the maternity hospital is ready to allow all this – [they] welcome [us]. [The hospital administration says:] "Yes, we will give the [baby's] body," "Yes, we will let everybody [parents] come." But they cannot, they don't have competences, time and resources to talk with parents.*
>
> (interview with the head of the NGO palliative care service)

She continued:

> *About the children's hospice, which is the basis for the perinatal palliative care program, we have approximately 200 children on lung ventilation (ALV) [at home]. I mean, we have recently discussed that if something happens with us as an organization, then the NICUs of Moscow will not cope. Because where would they place 200 people on ALV? No idea. This is a working system already.*
>
> (interview with the head of the NGO palliative care service)

The head of the service makes it clear that NGOs are working with the issues that remain uncovered by the maternity and healthcare system. They are more oriented to the requirements of beneficiaries (women and families) than to the bureaucratic needs of the State. They usually start as a response to demands from those who feel the most vulnerable within the maternity care system. Their beneficiaries expect actions that benefit *people*, not the State's bureaucracy and the System. Therefore, their ideas of "good care" are more oriented to the needs of women and families.

To become sustainable, such NGOs manage to get support and create shared meanings and practices with many other actors in the field. Among the outcomes of their activities are an orientation to targeted aid and to long-term systemic changes to implement "best practices." Paradoxically, they can challenge the System if they can get support from people who have high positions in this System and can influence maternity care policies. NGOs try to attract professionals who can work as engineers of change and create effective alliances. It helps to expand activities from targeted help toward systemic changes enshrined in administrative documents, educational and professional standards, and legislation. Successful cases, though rare, illustrate the prospects and feasibility of the advocated approaches. Not all NGOs become successful and sustainable, as they often face noticeable resistance from incumbents, and their development proceeds slowly and irregularly. But in certain cases, such as the one we have described earlier, they are effective in terms of changing the balance of power and becoming noticeable actors in the field of maternity care to challenge and change the existing rules and to formulate new ideas and practices of "good care."

Conclusion: care providers negotiating with/against the System

In Russia, professional power is mostly maintained along with State politics and loyalty to the System. However, as our research shows, despite ongoing changes in maternity care, both care providers and receivers are often not satisfied with the status quo. Both sides must systematically make many efforts in order to get their needs met, to maintain workable institutional conditions and to receive and provide "good care." However, providers can empower themselves by challenging existing rules and the institutional order. The challengers have to mobilize resources and supporters among professional communities and/or citizens, create alliances and become *political* in order to make improvements, however small and incremental they may be. All of our provider interlocutors referred to *the System* (healthcare, maternity care and, more broadly, the State as a whole), with which they try to negotiate or to oppose (such as independent trade unions), though both are very difficult for small groups of professional activists. Challengers have to overcome the resistance of incumbents, who are suspicious and reluctant to make changes and try out new ideas, seeking to preserve the status quo. As challengers need to create alliances with those who are more powerful and have more resources, they have to find supporters in governmental units of different levels, or in the maternity care units that are opposed to the System. They mostly act step-by-step; however, their results are strategically changing the systemic structural rules and conditions in maternity care for both care providers and receivers. In this way, all cases of grassroots initiatives become political. These actors, though on a very limited scale, transform the ideas and practices of "good care" toward more women-oriented care, broaden the options of choice for both professionals and patients and, consequently, often manage to empower them.

Note

1 In the previous recertification system, every medical practitioner had to take a several-months-long formal educational course once every 5 years to maintain their certification. Now, in a radical change, all medical practitioners, including midwives, must take part in short educational, practically-oriented courses that are conducted on a regular basis (Continuing Medical Education). For midwives, the goals of these courses are generally to improve their positions in maternity care and to make childbirth more humanized.

References

Arthur, N., & Collin, S. (2014). Counsellors, counselling, and social justice: The professional is political. *Canadian Journal of Counselling and Psychotherapy*, 48(3), 171–177. Available at: https://cjc-rcc.ucalgary.ca/article/view/61030.

Belooussova, E. (2002). The 'natural childbirth' movement in Russia: Self-representation strategies. *Anthropology of East Europe Review*, 20(1), 11–18.

Borozdina, E. (2014a). Jazyk Nauki I Jazyk Ljubvi: Legitimacija Nezavisimoj Akusherskoj [Language of science and language of love: The legitimation of independent Midwifery practice in Russia]. *Laboratorium*, 6(1), 30–59 (In Russian).

Borozdina, E. (2014b). Social'naja Organizacija Estestvennyh Rodov (Sluchaj Centra Akusherskogo Uhoda) [The social organization of natural childbirth (The case of center for Midwifery care)]. *Journal Of Social Policy Studies [Journal of Social Policy Studies]*, 12(3), 413–426. (In Russian)

Borozdina, E. (2017). Midwifery profession in Russia: Institutional context and everyday professional practices. *Medicina nei Secoli*, 29(4), 89–109.

Borozdina, E. (2018). Introducing 'natural' childbirth in Russian hospitals. Midwives' institutional work. In O. Zvonareva, E. Popova, & K. Horstman (Eds.), *Health, Technologies, and Politics in Post-Soviet Settings* (pp. 145–171). Cham: Palgrave Macmillan. https://doi.org/10.1007/978-3-319-64149-2_6.

Borozdina, E., & Novkunskaya, A. (2020). Patient-centered care in Russian maternity hospitals: Introducing a new approach through professionals' agency. *Health: An Interdisciplinary Journal for the Social Study of Health, Illness and Medicine*, 1–21. https://doi.org/10.1177/1363459320925871.

Davis-Floyd, R., & Johnson, C. B. (2006). *Mainstreaming Midwives: The Politics of Change*. New York: Routledge.

Edmonds, M. B. (2019). The professional is political: On citational practice and the persistent problem of academic plunder. *Journal of Feminist Scholarship*, 16(16).

Fligstein, N. (2008). *Theory and Methods for the Study of Strategic Action Fields*. Berkeley: University of California.

Fligstein, N., & McAdam, D. (2011). Toward a general theory of strategic action fields. *Sociological Theory*, 29, 1–26.

Hartman, A. (1993). The professional is political. *Social Work*, 38(4), 365–366, 504.

Hockey, J., & Draper, J. (2005). Beyond the womb and the tomb: Identity, (dis) embodiment and the life course. *Body & Society*, 11(2), 41–57.

Keane, H. (2009). Foetal personhood and representations of the absent child in pregnancy loss memorialization. *Feminist Theory*, 10(2), 153–171.

Layne, L. L. (2003). *Motherhood Lost: A Feminist Account of Pregnancy Loss in America*. London and New York: Routledge.

Leykin, I., & Rivkin-Fish, M. (2022). Politicized demography and biomedical authority in post-soviet Russia. *Medical Anthropology Theory*, in print.

Nakachi, M. (2021). *Replacing the Dead: The Politics of Reproduction in the Post-war Soviet Union*. Oxford and New York: Oxford University Press.

Novkunskaya, A. (2018). Bjudzhetnye Gospital'nye Rody V Rossijskoj Sisteme Zdravoohranenija: Razlichija V Podhodah [State-funded facility-based childbirth in the Russian system of healthcare: Diversity of approaches]. *Antropologicheskij forum [Anthropological Forum]*, 37, 177–197. http://doi.org/10.31250/1815-8870-2018-14-37-177-197 (In Russian).

Novkunskaya, A. (2020). *Professional Agency and Institutional Change: Case of Maternity Services in Small-Town Russia*. Doctoral thesis, University of Helsinki.

Odent, M. (1984). *Birth Reborn*. Glasgow: William Collins Sons & Co, Ltd.

Ozhiganova, A. A. (2019a). 'What do women want': Motives of refusal of maternity hospital in favor of home birth. *Monitoring of Public Opinion: Economic and Social Changes*, 2, 263–281. https://doi.org/10.14515/monitoring.2019.2.12.

Ozhiganova, A. A. (2019b). Oficial'noe (biomedicinskoe) i al'ternativnoe (domashnee) akusherstvo. Praktiki formalizovannogo i neformal'nogo vzaimodejstvija [Official (biomedical) obstetrics and alternative (home) Midwifery: Formalized and informal interaction practices]. *Jekonomicheskaja sociologija [Journal of Economic Sociology]*, 20(5), 28–52 (In Russian).

Ozhiganova, A. A. (2019c). Istorija rossijskogo dvizhenija za domashnie rody i osoznannoe roditel'stvo (1980-e gody–nastojashhee vremja) [The history of Russian movement for homebirth and attachment parenting (from 1980s to present time)]. *Medical Anthropology and Bioethics*, 17(1) (In Russian).

Ozhiganova, A. A. (2020). Avtoritetnoe znanie o rodah i rodovspomozhenii: analiz diskursivnyh praktik rossijskih perinatal'nyh specialistov [Authoritative knowledge of childbirth and obstetrics: Analysis of discursive practices of Russian perinatal specialists]. *Population and Economics*, 4(4), 84–99. https://doi.org/10.3897/popecon.4.e57267 (In Russian).

Ozhiganova, A. A. (2021). Trud Douly, Publichnyj I Intimnyj: Professional'naja Zabota, Samoorga-Nizacija I Aktivizm [Doula's work, public and intimate: Professional care, self-organization and activism]. *Monitoring of Public Opinion: Economic and Social Changes*, 3, 200–225. https://doi.org/10.14515/monitoring.2021.3.1903 (In Russian).

Rossiter, A. (2000). The professional is political: An interpretation of the problem of the past in solution-focused therapy. *American Journal of Orthopsychiatry*, 70(2), 150–161. https://doi.org/10.1037/h0087656.

Starobinets, A. A. (2017). *Posmotri na nego [Look at Him]*. Moscow: Corpus.

Conclusions

Struggling with and within the System for "good" maternity care

In this book we asked and answered the following questions: What constitutes "good maternity care" in Russia in the 21st century? Why, after numerous reforms and improvements, does maternity care in Russia continue to underserve the interests of its providers and receivers? How do actors in the field of maternity care struggle for "good care" in their routine interactions within maternity hospitals and beyond? And how does "political" correspond with "professional" in this field of struggle?

The notion of "good care" in Russian maternity care is not constant nor consistent, but rather an issue of negotiation. Global neoliberal tendencies, along with the Soviet legacy and the post-Soviet reforms of maternity care, have resulted in notable changes in the care practices and ideals of both medical providers and receivers. Maternity care has become a field of struggle among different actors – healthcare providers (obstetricians, neonatologists, midwives, nurses, hospital administrators, etc.), the market, childbearing women, NGOs and professional alliances and the State/the System – all of these have different spheres of interest and differing ideals of "good care."

In this book, among other issues, we have placed primary focus on the arrangements and maternity care provision of Russian maternity hospitals – the only legal institutions for maternity care provision in Russia. We conducted our primary ethnographic research in one large Level 3 hospital, which we have called "the Hospital" herein. As we conducted our research in the Hospital, we continually reflected on the question of what it means to do ethnographic research in a relatively closed medical facility in Russia, full of negotiations among different actors, including ourselves. We had to continually perform our positioning and work to engender trust in ourselves – to establish ourselves not as outside Others, but as insiders belonging to *svoi* ("our people"), as "sociologists in white" who came to form a part of the Hospital community. Different interlocutors in different wards constantly examined and questioned our positionality within the Hospital, and we equally constantly explained who we are and what we were doing there. Moreover, we still continue to prove our relevance, as more than three years after we exited this field, we maintain varying levels of cooperation with our

DOI: 10.4324/9781003139539-7

interlocutors: they invite us to give presentations at their conferences and to share their current plans and ideas, and we participate in joint follow-up projects. Here we outline the five major conclusions we have reached as a result of the research we conducted for this book.

Conclusion #1. Maternity care as part of a hybrid System: rule-following and care discontinuities

Our first conclusion relates to maternity care as *the System*. Our research has shown that "the System" is a hybrid of Soviet bureaucratic paternalism and post-Soviet neoliberal managerialism and marketization. Despite the reforms of the last decades and the growing market competitiveness that have provoked changes, Russian maternity care remains highly medicalized and centralized. Different logics of regulation emerge simultaneously and evoke inconsistencies in rules and standards, which in turn result in discontinuities of care. The State acts in a paternalistic way as the main regulator, implementing its own bureaucratic criteria for "good care" – the kind of care that presupposes the total accountability of maternity care providers (via endless paperwork) – and that is oriented toward achieving targeted indicators for births, neonatal and maternal deaths, abortions and other demographically significant indicators.

At the same time, hospitals have to follow the neoliberal rules and, thus, are expected to be financially efficient and attract more patients to remain sustainable. This means that they have to offer competitive service for their clients/patients, meet their needs, and provide opportunities for choice. These contradict the State's demand for paternalistic obedience – obstetricians and other physicians are supposed to be authoritative experts who subordinate patients, and in turn are subordinated by confusing and contradictory State, hospital and departmental rules and regulations. Neither physicians nor midwives nor childbearing women are satisfied with this situation, as it limits the possibilities for patient-centered "good care" and the professional autonomy of maternity care providers. The other meaning of the System (of health and maternity care) is its distancing and alienation from the needs of both providers and patients and orientation to State bureaucratic demands. Here we remind our readers of the statement made by a midwife interlocutor: this is "*the System, where is nobody is interested in a woman and a newborn . . . the System put me in a cage.*"

Conclusion # 2. The positioning of childbearing women in the Russian hybrid system of maternity care: individualistic orientations

Our second conclusion is related *to the positioning of childbearing women* in this hybrid system. In Soviet maternity care, women had no choice, were vulnerable and experienced a great deal of suffering in industrialized, conveyer-like maternity hospitals. Nowadays, pregnant women have many more opportunities as consumers, but are not empowered as citizens, and still have no channels for collective influence on the quality of biomedical maternity care or the State politics and policies related to this care.

As clients, many women have become more assertive – they spend a lot of time and make multiple efforts to organize and negotiate "good care" during pregnancy and childbirth in medical settings, looking for the "right choice" among the available options. As clients, they want their personal needs to be taken into account, including their expectations of better service and comfort, along with high-quality medical help and more emotional support from providers. However, the choices they do have are limited, as birth occurs mostly in State-funded hospitals; homebirth and independent midwifery practice are illegal (though they do exist on a small scale); and private maternity hospitals are rare and financially unaffordable for most.

Therefore, women's strategies are individualistically oriented; they try to personalize relations with obstetricians and midwives by carefully choosing and, officially or informally, paying them in order to receive more personalized and humanistic care. Yet this care is still organized in a mostly paternalistic way. In other words, the strategy of care personalization often doesn't work well in the System, which, in its pronatalist bent, is interested in improving maternity care. Maternity care is highly oriented to the State's strict bureaucratic demands, and this orientation leads to the discontent of care receivers. While possibilities for better care in Russian maternity hospitals are limited by structural conditions, women blame individual providers for inappropriate clinical actions, lack of comfort and emotional support, and rudeness. As consumers, they have instruments for channeling their discontent: they can complain to official State bodies and on social media if they do not receive "good care." Yet their struggle for "good care" remains oriented to individual good, not to the collective good. The growing number of discontents and complaints, which care providers mostly find unfair, leads to situations in which healthcare providers and receivers appear to be "on different sides of the barricade."

Conclusion #3. The contradictory structural positions of maternity care providers: trapped "between a rock and a hard place"

Our third conclusion highlights the contradictory structural positions of maternity care providers. They lack professional autonomy, feel increasing regulatory pressure from the State (via bureaucracy and threats of punishment) and experience a different kind of pressure from women's growing consumeristic demands – in other words, as the saying goes, they are "trapped between a rock and a hard place." We obtained seemingly endless evidence that maternity care practitioners try to provide the best care they can, but their possibilities are limited by the numerous, often contradictory, bureaucratic and economic requirements imposed on them. They feel themselves vulnerable and alienated under overall control and contradictory demands from the State and from their patients.

In order to make local conditions workable, providers have to accomplish not only clinical tasks, but also extra-clinical work, acting as service providers, State bureaucrats, effective managers, psychotherapists, etc. Practitioners make many personal efforts to do their best in settings of inconsistent yet strictly obligatory rules. They *manually manage* inconsistencies – that is, they personally negotiate and coordinate professional activities in the grey areas in-between official rules. Such informal coordination is needed to manage numerous both routine and urgent problems when official rules are unclear and unhelpful.

In addition to the State rules, every maternity care facility or ward works out a specific set of local rules, maintaining them differentially, and this creates even more institutional inconsistencies and organizational gaps between different facilities, leading to discontinuity of care. When women face different rules in different wards and facilities and receive contradictory recommendations from different obstetricians and other physicians, their discontent increases. In order to ameliorate this discontent and prevent consumer complaints, providers increase the volume of their emotional labor and change their emotional styles. The formerly taken-for-granted Soviet *khamstvo* gives way to more client-oriented communicative practices, such as politeness and smiling; and certainly, this change is beneficial for patients. However, *khamstvo* remains one of the instruments of disciplining childbearing women and fitting them into the institutional order, while providers juggle the different emotional tools of politeness and rudeness, using smiling and kind words to cajole laboring women into doing what their care providers want them to, and *khamstvo* when such women do not comply. Within these conditions, providers try to use best practices, but their activities mostly bring only here-and-now benefits for individual women and do not result in systemic changes, because they do not challenge the existent institutional order (the System) nor their own positions within it.

Conclusion #4. Providers' agencies and voices: the professional as political

Our fourth conclusion is about the *voice and agency* of those professionals who challenge the existing System, contribute to the humanistic improvement of maternity care and empower both its providers and receivers. We argue that in such cases, *professional issues become political.* New semi-legal attendants such as doulas; hospital midwives and nurses; obstetricians; professional associations; allies in administration and ruling bodies, independent trade unions; and NGOs are among the System's challengers. Challengers initiate struggles *for* professional autonomy and better care, and *against* the System and its incumbents. The repertoire of their strategies ranges from mostly invisible actions on the ground level to the promotion of new educational programs and professional standards, and making political statements. In challenging existing rules, challengers face considerable resistance from incumbents who wish to preserve the institutional status quo; therefore, their actions require strong personal commitment and can be risky. The changes that they bring start slowly and locally; their influence on the national level is usually quite limited, but in some cases, over time they come to constitute the avant-garde of their professional communities, successfully filling the gaps in the State-funded maternity care System, to the extent that they become notable agents in the field.

Conclusion #5. Gender and Paternalism in Russian Maternity Care

A feminist approach has been important in our study; thus, our fifth conclusion is related to the gendered dimension of maternity care. Neo-traditionalism, pronatalist State politics and the current concept of "intensive mothering" in Russia are important contexts for maternity care provision. However, the limitations on the provision of "good care" cannot be explained by patriarchy only. *Paternalism* as an institutional power is no less important in Russia than patriarchy. In Russian paternalism, women expect the State, maternity care facilities as State institutions, and obstetricians as State representatives to have the authority to manage the perinatal process in multiple ways, caring for dependent women from the top down.

Most obstetricians and almost all midwives in Russia are women, yet they show little to no interest in feministic solidarity, as they remain incumbents trying to maintain their medicalized power and hierarchical authoritative positions, and to support the existing institutional order. As noted here, many care receivers also look for paternalistic instead of egalitarian or empowering relations with providers; *consumeristic paternalism* satisfies their needs. In Russia, some female patients and practitioners benefit from neoliberal reforms in maternity care: the former have more choice and receive better care (especially if they pay for it), while the latter get better working conditions and financial benefits.

However, we have observed some feminist reflections both among providers (some midwives and doulas call themselves feminists) and childbearing women – as feminism has become more popular in Russia in recent years, though it still causes suspicions and tensions with more conservative social groups. Along with feminism, the State bureaucracy (the System) becomes a common issue for critique, as it produces many inconsistencies and barriers to dialogue between care providers and receivers, and consequently impedes the emergence of shared ideals of "good care."

The multiple meanings of "good care" in the Russian maternity care context

We conclude this book with a comprehensive overview of what "good care" actually is, or is thought to be, in Russian maternity care. As a result of our study, we have come to the conclusion that "good care" in Russian maternity hospitals appears not solely as a project of "women's empowerment," but rather springs from the complex of negotiations among different actors in the limited opportunities of institutional settings. For the State, "good care" is the strict following of top-down rules and getting "proper" indicators for childbirth, health, and mortality. For hospital-based maternity care providers (and especially for obstetricians and those in administrative positions), "good care" is a confusing concept – they should follow the State rules and professional standards for "good care," whereas at the same time they are to be economically effective, attract more patients and money, and should do their work professionally, while taking into account the expectations of childbearing women, including their needs for emotional support and more humanistic care. "Good care" for these practitioners, including obstetricians, constitutes an assemblage of the State's and clients' demands, which they try to meet in the settings of limited resources, contradictory rules and local circumstances. In order to get closer to this notion in practice, they manually manage this contradictory care, adapting it to each specific setting and particular case.

Obstetricians take the entire responsibility for childbirth and "good care" in Russia, and, thus, maternity care is highly medicalized. It is supposed by the State orders and designs of maternity care institutions that midwives should just follow instructions and assist physicians; however, in some cases, midwives claim more agency and promote a less medicalized and more humanistic approach. Obstetricians are now oriented toward providing more (superficially) humanistic, but still medicalized, standardized and paternalistic care. (We note here that Davis-Floyd (2018) distinguishes between "superficial" and "deep" humanism – in the latter, care is fully individualized; in the former, it is not.) In commercial departments offering paid services, "good care" presupposes more emotional labor and attention to women's needs, and more flexibility in approaches to childbirth; this trend is gradually permeating other departments.

For independent and semi-independent attendants, "good care" is more oriented toward women's expectations, but these attendants are restricted in the amount of resources available to them, and lack legal status. For some activists among obstetricians, other physicians, and midwives, "good care" can be achieved only via comprehensive structural changes in the System; thus, they try to struggle for such changes, which, as they claim, enhance the possibility to provide and receive "good care." For childbearing women, "good care" means receiving attentive care in a polite manner, as opposed to the Soviet factory-line approach and communicative style of *khamstvo*. They have become demanding, voicing their discontent; they want their (multiple and various) expectations about childbirth to be met. Those who can afford it are often ready to pay for this kind of "good care"; however, again, they mostly opt for "consumeristic paternalism" – in other words, for paternalistic, yet individualized, service as the most beneficial for them and their babies.

These multiple definitions of "good care" demonstrate that there is no consensus about what constitutes it among the multiple actors in Russian maternity care; rather, each group mentioned here has its own definition of "good care." To briefly summarize, for the State, "good care" means reformation of the System, improvements in its quality and conformity, financial and technical self-sufficiency and, most importantly, the top-down elaboration of the rules that practitioners should follow. For hospital administrators, "good care" means following State rules while being economically effective; for obstetricians, it means providing medicalized and paternalistic, yet also more humanistic care (in comparison with Soviet maternity care). For those offering paid care, "good care" means flexibility and more variations in the kind of care offered, often less medicalization and more attention to women's needs; for childbearing women, "good care" generally means a combination of paternalistic *and* personalized "good" services.

These conflicting definitions of "good care" reflect the conflicting desires and goals of these multiple actors and culminate in the tensions they place on the most responsible parties – obstetricians and midwives. Thus, again, these care providers are placed between "a rock and a hard place" – meaning the pressures on obstetricians to provide what other, more authoritative State bodies conceive of as "good care" by following the standardized rules; obstetricians' own definitions of (medicalized, paternalistic, humanistic) "good care"; and women's desires for what they conceive of as (consumeristic, paternalistic, humanistic, individualized) "good care." The similarities (paternalistic, humanistic) between these definitions can result in women's sense that they did receive "good care"; the differences (medicalized vs. consumeristic and individualized) can result in women's perceptions that they did not receive "good care." Women know in advance about the risks of dissatisfaction and believe that if they pay for less medicalized care, they can switch from a patient to a consumer – although in practice, even if women pay, their expectations of "good care" are not necessarily fulfilled. The win-win here could stem from less medicalized and more individualized obstetric care – but that "win-win" could also result in obstetricians' penalization for not following the rules of the System – the "rock and the hard place" described earlier. This metaphor also characterizes much of the Russian maternity care system, as we have sought to show in this volume for the practitioners of the Hospital.

We have also sought to show how numerous post-Soviet top-down reforms have led to inconsistent yet rigid rules in maternity care. Providers – first of all, obstetricians and hospital administrators – have to navigate patients into the System *manually* on a daily basis, as the State and childbearing women have different demands, expectations and ideas about "good care." All parties have to adapt, individually or in negotiations, their strategies in this inconsistent, hybrid system. Actors blame each other if something goes wrong; only few of them resist collectively, blaming the System and calling for radical changes. Ultimately, in this book, we have sought to provide a detailed overview and analysis of the hybridization of post-Soviet maternity care and its effects on administrators, practitioners and women, which we studied in the Hospital as "sociologists in white."

References

Davis-Floyd, R. (2018). The technocratic, humanistic, and holistic paradigms of birth and health care. In R. Davis-Floyd (Ed.), *Ways of Knowing about Birth: Mothers, Midwives, Medicine, and Birth Activism* (pp. 3–44). Long Grove IL: Waveland Press.

Appendices

Appendix I

Qualitative data on challengers of the maternity care system (2021)

Short description: This dataset contains qualitative data from different projects and single interviews. We picked the sources that referred to the "challengers" of maternity care system, described in Chapter 6. Some data was collected specifically for this chapter.

Researchers: A. Temkina, D. Litvina, A. Novkunskaya.

Case 1. Hospital midwives struggling for "good care": from informalities to professional associations

Data for this case consist of two focus groups with midwives 2020–2021, one interview in 2015 and observations at numerous workshops and conferences 2017–2019. This research was conducted with the support of the Anna Temkina Professorship on Health and Gender.

Case 2. Activists and an independent trade union struggling for "good care": public voices and the case of Hospital M.

Data for this case consist of one interview with a midwife (2021), two interviews with Deputy Chairmans of the trade union (2019, 2021), document analysis of media publications related to the case since 2016 and the normative acts and State orders (2021). This research was conducted with the support of the Anna Temkina Professorship on Health and Gender.

Case 3. NGOs struggling for "good care": the case of perinatal palliative care

Data for this case consist of 20 interviews with professionals who interact with women in situations of reproductive loss (stillbirth, miscarriage): psychologists, physicians (obstetricians, neonatologists, specialists in diagnostics), midwives, doulas. Among them, 12 are related to the NGOs, working *in* them or *with* them. We also rely on observations in hospitals and field notes made on medical professional events (workshops, conferences). We conducted this research from 2018 to 2021 with the support of the Russian Science Foundation (grant N 19-78-10128).

Appendix 2

Interviews with patients of the Hospital (2020)

Name of the project: Patient-centered care in Russian healthcare: organizational challenges and professionals' opportunities (2020).

Funding: This research was conducted with the support of the Russian Science Foundation (grant N 19-78-10128).

Short description: This dataset includes 15 semi-structured interviews with women, who (or whose infants) received pre-, intra- or postnatal medical care in the Hospital in recent years, and one extra interview with a woman who was getting gynecological and surgical healthcare services and shared with us her Soviet birth experience (Zina). The duration of these interviews varied from 26 to 190 minutes. The goal was to analyze women's experiences in communication and encounters with maternity care providers.

Researchers: A. Temkina (head), D. Litvina, T. Loboda, A. Novkunskaya, M. Vyatchina.

#	*Pseudonym*	*Gender*	*Type of medical help that a woman received in the Hospital, covered by, year:*	*Age (at time of interview)*
1	Alla	Female	Delivery (second child), covered by medical insurance, 2018	30
2	Valeria	Female	Neonatal surgery and further rehabilitation (second child), covered by medical insurance, 2016	36
3	Lilia	Female	Delivery (only child), paid service, 2019	29
4	Nina	Female	Delivery (both children), covered by medical insurance, 2016, 2018	29
5	Polina	Female	Prenatal consultations, delivery (both children), covered by medical insurance, 2016, 2019	43

(Continued)

(Continued)

#	*Pseudonym*	*Gender*	*Type of medical help that a woman received in the Hospital, covered by, year:*	*Age (at time of interview)*
6	Anna	Female	Delivery (only child), covered by medical insurance, 2016. Rehabilitation twice a year since 2017	32
7	Elvira	Female	Delivery (only child) and maternal surgery, covered by medical insurance, 2017	38
8	Irina	Female	Prenatal consultations, delivery (only child), covered by medical insurance, paid extra services (personal room), 2017	32
9	Alisa	Female	Delivery (only child), covered by medical insurance, 2016. Surgery for child, 2017	32
10	Veronika	Female	Prenatal medical aid and delivery (only child), covered by medical insurance, 2019	22
11	Vlada	Female	Prenatal consultations, delivery (second child), covered by medical insurance, 2019	35
12	Maria	Female	Delivery (second child), paid service, 2019	31
13	Anastasia	Female	Delivery (only child) and further long period in neonatal resuscitation unit, covered by medical insurance, 2018	33
14	Diana	Female	Prenatal consultations (unofficial), delivery (first child), covered by medical insurance, 2013	36
15	Nadezhda	Female	Delivery (only child), covered by medical insurance, 2020	27
16	Zina	Female	Delivery (only child), covered by medical insurance, 1989	56

Appendix 3

Ethnography in the Hospital (2019)

Name of the project: Patient-centered care in Russian healthcare: organizational challenges and professionals' opportunities (2019).

Funding: This research was conducted with the support of the Russian Science Foundation (grant N 19-78-10128).

Short description: This dataset includes details on ethnographic sessions within the Hospital, conducted in 2019. The goals were to study communications within and between medical departments, to analyze how patients' complaints and discontents were being formed in the maternity care facility and to describe how the organization of continuity of care (and emerging institutional gaps) shaped the patients' childbirth experiences.

Researchers: A. Temkina (head), D. Litvina, A. Novkunskaya.

#	*Researcher*	*Duration (hrs)*	*Field site(s)*	*Number of pages in Field Diary*
1	Anna Temkina	6	9.15–9.40: Conference hall (morning conference); 10.00–16.00: Ward of pathological pregnancy (prenatal ward)	6
2	Daria Litvina	6.5	9.25–9.40: Conference hall (morning conference); 10.00–16.00: Ward of pathological pregnancy (prenatal ward)	10.5
3	Anastasia Novkunskaya	4	9.15–9.40: Ward of pathological pregnancy (prenatal ward) 10.00–12.45: Office of the chief nurse	5
4	Anna Temkina	7.5	9.30–11.00: Office of the head of the Hospital (and the corridor while waiting for audience) 11.00–17.00: Emergency room	7

(Continued)

(Continued)

#	*Researcher*	*Duration (hrs)*	*Field site(s)*	*Number of pages in Field Diary*
5	Daria Litvina	7.5	9.30–11.00: Office of the head of the Hospital (and the corridor while waiting for audience) 11.00–17.00: Emergency room	12
6	Anna Temkina	9	9.30–18.00: Reception	12
7	Daria Litvina	6.5	9.00–10.00: Parking (facilities for patients) 10.10–16.30: Reception	14
8	Anastasia Novkunskaya	8	9.30–15.00: Following the chief nurse 15.10–17.30: Department of consultation and diagnostics	11
9	Anna Temkina	8	9.30–16.40: Department of consultation and diagnostics 17.10–17.30: Office of the head of the Hospital	10
10	Daria Litvina	7.5	9.30–16.40: Department of consultation and diagnostics 17.10–17.30: Office of the head of the Hospital	16
11	Anastasia Novkunskaya	6.5	9.40–10.20: Conference hall 10.20–12.15: Office of the chief nurse 12.15–13.50: Reception (evacuation because of a telephone call about a terroristic attack) 13.40–16.10: Office of the chief nurse	14
12	Anastasia Novkunskaya	6.5	9.30–11.20: Conference hall (morning conference) 11.20–15.25: Office of the chief nurse 15.25–16.10: Reception (evacuation)	7
13	Anastasia Novkunskaya	8	9.10–9.45: Conference hall 9.45–13.25: Office of the chief nurse 13.25–14.45: Lunch in the main building 14.45–16.45: Cabinet of the chief nurse, corridor	10
14	Anna Temkina	7.5	10.00–11.45: Administrative floor (chief nurse, corridor, cabinet of the head doctor) 11.50–17.20: Postnatal ward, Department of Physiology and Pathology of Newborn, Lunch with staff psychologists in the main building	9
15	Daria Litvina	7.5	10.00–11.45: Administrative floor (chief nurse, corridor, cabinet of the head doctor) 11.50–17.20: Postnatal ward, Department of Physiology and Pathology of Newborn, Lunch with staff psychologists in the main building	16

#	*Researcher*	*Duration (hrs)*	*Field site(s)*	*Number of pages in Field Diary*
16	Anastasia Novkunskaya	5	13.00–17.30: Office of the chief nurse 17.30–18.00: Reception	4.5
17	Anna Temkina	9.5	9.30–9.50: Office of the head of the Hospital 10.10–19.00: Department of Resuscitation	10
18	Daria Litvina	9.5	9.30–9.50: Office of the head of the Hospital 10.10–19.00: Department of Resuscitation	20
19	Anastasia Novkunskaya	4	14.10–18.10: Following the chief nurse	10
20	Daria Litvina	9.5	09.15–09.40: Conference hall 09.50–18.20: The Department of Newborn Physiology	21
21	Anna Temkina	9.5	09.15–09.40: Conference hall 09.50–18.20: The Department of Newborn Physiology	14
22	Anastasia Novkunskaya	7	09.20–16.20: Following the chief nurse	7
23	Anna Temkina	10.5	9.15–9.35: Conference hall 10.00–18.30: Department of Newborn Pathology 18.30–19.40: Office of the head of the Hospital	17
24	Daria Litvina	9.6	10.00–18.30: Department of Newborn Pathology 18.30–19.40: Office of the head of the Hospital	17
25	Anna Temkina	9	9.15–9.40: Conference hall 9.40–10.10: Corridor (next to printing station) 10 15–18.15: Following the head doctor (NICU/Neonatal Intensive Care Unit; Perinatal Consilium consists of multi-disciplinary team of medical professionals and is aimed at working out tactics of further treatment in complicated medical cases	19
26	Anna Temkina	7.5	11.00–Talking with the head doctor 11.20–18.20: Emergency room 12.40–13.40: Department of Telemedicine 16.40–17.20: Express laboratory	13
27	Daria Litvina	7	11.00–Talking with the head doctor 11.20–18.20: Emergency room and 12.40–13.40: Department of Telemedicine 16.40–17.20: Express laboratory	13

(*Continued*)

(Continued)

#	*Researcher*	*Duration (hrs)*	*Field site(s)*	*Number of pages in Field Diary*
28	Anna Temkina	8.5	10.30–19.12: Department of Child Surgery	9
29	Daria Litvina	8.5	10.30–19.12: Department of Child Surgery	11
30	Anna Temkina	9	19.00–4.00: Delivery ward	12
31	Daria Litvina	9	19.00–4.00: Delivery ward	15
32	Anna Temkina	5	13.10–16.45: Office of the head of the Hospital 16.45–18.00: Dining room	12
33	Daria Litvina	5	13.10–16.45: Office of the head of the Hospital 16.45–18.00: Dining room	7
	Total	249		391

Appendix 4

Interviews with health practitioners and patients of the Hospital (2018)

Name of the project: Medical interactions in the changing childbirth services: women's needs and professionals' opportunities (2018)

Funding: This research was conducted with the support of the Anna Temkina Professorship on Health and Gender.

Short description: This research aimed to investigate how patients' complaints and discontents were being formed in the Hospital and how the organization of care continuity (and emerging institutional gaps) shaped the patients' childbirth experiences. The research data consist of a series of observations in the Hospital, in-depth semi-structured interviews with the Hospital workers – administrators, physicians, nurses and midwives (n = 19), in-depth interviews with patients in prenatal and postpartum units (n = 8) and document analysis (official complaints, online reports on the Internet, n = 35) (more detailed on media reviews – in Appendix 5).

Researchers: A. Temkina (head), A. Novkunskaya

#	*Pseudonym*	*Gender*	*Position within the Hospital*
1–2	Irina Nikolaevna	Female	Chief physician
3	Elena Vladimirovna	Female	MD, Director of the Hospital
4	Oleg Borisovich	Male	MD, Director of the Hospital
5–6	Jurii	Male	Head of department
7	Valentina	Female	Head of department
8	Anzhelika	Female	Midwife
9	Mila	Female	Head of department
10	Olga	Female	Midwife
11	Anastasia	Female	Midwife
12	Vladimir Mikhailovich	Male	Head of department
13	Innokenty	Male	Head of department
14	Alla Nikolaevna	Female	Chief midwife of the Hospital

(Continued)

(Continued)

#	*Pseudonym*	*Gender*	*Position within the Hospital*
15	Irina Petrovna	Female	Main midwife of a perinatal ward
16	Olga Borisovna	Female	Midwife of prenatal ward
17	Elena Petrovna	Female	Midwife of prenatal ward
18	Anna Alekseevna	Female	Midwife of prenatal ward
19	Varvara Alekseevna	Female	Head of department

#	*Pseudonym*	*Gender*	*Position within the Hospital*	*Age*
20	Antonina	Female	Patient of prenatal ward	40
21	Alina	Female	Patient of prenatal ward	35
22	Elena	Female	Patient of prenatal ward	39
23	Olga	Female	Patient of prenatal ward	32
24	Nina	Female	Patient of prenatal ward	27
25	Elizaveta	Female	Patient of postnatal ward	23
26	Ekaterina	Female	Patient of postnatal ward	27
27	Galina	Female	Patient of prenatal ward	40

Appendix 5

Media reviews of the Hospital (2018)

Short description: Analysis of the reviews posted on one of the most well-known parenting forums – "Little one" – written by parents (predominantly mothers) on the Hospital's maternity services, which they received in the Hospital 2011–2018.

Out of 138 posts overall, 35 ranked the services quite low (1–3 "stars" out of 5) and contained complaints and expressions of discontent. Those posts were selected and analyzed along with the general structure

Researchers: A. Temkina (head), A. Novkunskaya

Appendix 6

Posts in social media with the hashtag #nasilievrodah ("violence in childbirth") (2018–2019)

Short description: Analysis of online posts with the hashtag #nasilievrodah ("violence in childbirth"). Concurrent online community was (created 11th November 2016 in social network VKontakte (vk.com/humanize_birth). At the time of analysis it had 12,465 subscribers and 860 posts (Accessed 23.09.2018). Data included into detailed analysis:

- 30 posts made 21 October 2016–13 November 2016;
- 20 posts, made 29 November 2017–17 February 2018;
- Interview with moderator.

Researcher: A. Temkina

Appendix 7

Interviews with women who paid for maternity services (2015–2016)

Name of the project: Health, Choice, and Paid Service in Maternity Care (2015–2016)

Funding: This research was conducted with the support of the Anna Temkina Professorship on Health and Gender.

Short description: The goal of the project was to analyze what maternity hospitals offer for purchase, how women make their choices and what are their demands and their reasons for paying for services that are available for free. This dataset includes semi-structured interviews (n=35) with women who gave birth after 2012 in Russian maternity care facilities and paid for services, and one extra interview with Zhenya, an obstetrician aged 52.

Researchers: A. Temkina (head), E. Borozdina (coordinator), H. Akhundzade, M. Godovannya, E. Ivanova, D. Khodorenko, A. Ugarova, A. Klimova, D. Zhaivoronok.

#	*Pseudonym*	*Gender*	*Number of children*	*Age (at the time of interview)*
1	Viktoria	Female	One child	28
2	Alia	Female	One child	29
3	Maria	Female	One child	26
4	Regina	Female	One child	35
5	Lida	Female	One child	26
6	Inna	Female	One child	34
7	Yaroslava	Female	One child	30
8	Alena	Female	One child	27
9	Marta	Female	Two children	31
10	Nina	Female	One child	37
11	Evdokiya	Female	Three children	32
12	Olesya	Female	One child	40
13	Oksana	Female	Two children	35

(Continued)

(Continued)

#	*Pseudonym*	*Gender*	*Number of children*	*Age (at the time of interview)*
14	Tatjiana	Female	One child	28
15	Alexandra	Female	Two children	30
16	Ira	Female	One child	40
17	Tamara	Female	Three children	44
18	Oxana	Female	One child	27
19	Asya	Female	One child	31
20	Bella	Female	One child	32
21	Agrafena	Female	One child	30
22	Svetlana	Female	One child	20
23	Marina	Female	One child	25
24	Tais	Female	Two children	30
25	Zhanna	Female	One child	38
26	Emma	Female	One child	27
27	Sonya	Female	Four children	32
28	Julia	Female	One child	34
29	Nonna	Female	One child	29
30	Nina	Female	One child	29
31	Klavdia	Female	One child	27
32	Varja	Female	One child	27
33	Arina	Female	One child	27
34	Zoya	Female	Two children	28
35	Agata	Female	Two children	31
36	Zhenya	Female	An obstetrician	52

Appendix 8

Interviews with women who received maternity services for free (covered by mandatory health insurance) (2016–2017)

Name of the project: Choice, control and trust in childbirth (2016–2017)

Funding: This research was conducted with the support of the Anna Temkina Professorship on Health and Gender.

Short description: This dataset includes semi-structured interviews (n = 24) with women who gave birth after 2013 in State-funded facilities and did not pay for maternity services (they were covered by general Medical Health Insurance). The goal of the project was to analyze what are the practices of young women who receive free medical services in a large city. The research aimed to reveal whether choice is possible in free-of-charge care, and whether or not such women could exercise control during childbirth.

Researchers: A. Temkina (head), A. Novkunskaya (coordinator), E. Ivanova, D. Khodorenko, A. Savchenko, E. Tokalova, A. Ugarova, V. Zemenkov.

#	*Pseudonym*	*Gender*	*Number of children, year(s) of childbirth*	*Age (at the time of interview)*
1	Ariana	Female	One child	25
2	Evgeniya	Female	One child	30
3	Larisa	Female	One child`	30
4	Aleksandra	Female	One child	30
5	Vladislava	Female	One child	27
6	Arina	Female	One child	27
7	Anna	Female	One child	27
8	Vera	Female	Four children	33
9	Tatiana	Female	One child	26
10	Ekaterina	Female	One child	28
11	Rita	Female	One child	35
12	Maria	Female	Two children	28

(Continued)

(Continued)

#	*Pseudonym*	*Gender*	*Number of children, year(s) of childbirth*	*Age (at the time of interview)*
13	Alina	Female	One child	37
14	Ksenia	Female	One child	30
15	Tatiana	Female	Two children	28
16	Tamara	Female	Three children	33
17	Kamilya	Female	One child	32
18	Arina	Female	Two children	37
19	Kira	Female	Three children	33
20	Giulietta	Female	Four children	37
21	Ekaterina	Female	Six children	41
22	Miroslava	Female	One child	32
23	Margarita	Female	One child	28
24	Natalia	Female	One child	23

Index